5th Edition

Critical Thinking and Writing in Nursing

Bob Price

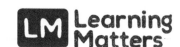

Learning Matters

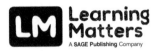

Learning Matters
A SAGE Publishing Company
1 Oliver's Yard
55 City Road
London EC1Y 1SP

SAGE Publications Inc.
2455 Teller Road
Thousand Oaks, California 91320

SAGE Publications India Pvt Ltd
B 1/I 1 Mohan Cooperative Industrial Area
Mathura Road
New Delhi 110 044

SAGE Publications Asia-Pacific Pte Ltd
3 Church Street
#10-04 Samsung Hub
Singapore 049483

First edition published 2010
Second edition 2013
Third edition 2016
Fourth edition 2019
Fifth edition 2021

Editor: Laura Walmsley
Development editor: Sarah Turpie
Senior project editor: Chris Marke
Project management: River Editorial
Marketing manager: George Kimble
Cover design: Wendy Scott
Typeset by: C&M Digitals (P) Ltd, Chennai, India
Printed in the UK

Library of Congress Control Number: 2020949580

British Library Cataloguing in Publication data

A catalogue record for this book is available from the British Library

ISBN 978-1-5297-2882-8
ISBN 978-1-5297-2881-1 (pbk)

Contents

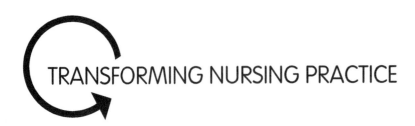

TRANSFORMING NURSING PRACTICE

Transforming Nursing Practice is a series tailor made for pre-registration student nurses. Each book in the series is:

 Affordable

 Mapped to the NMC Standards of proficiency for registered nurses

 Full of active learning features

 Focused on applying theory to practice

Each book addresses a core topic and they have been carefully developed to be simple to use, quick to read and written in clear language.

An invaluable series of books that explicitly relates to the NMC standards. Each book covers a different topic that students need to explore in order to develop into a qualified nurse... I would recommend this series to all Pre-Registered nursing students whatever their field or year of study.

LINDA ROBSON,
Senior Lecturer at Edge Hill University

Many titles in the series are on our recommended reading list and for good reason - the content is up to date and easy to read. These are the books that actually get used beyond training and into your nursing career.

EMMA LYDON,
Adult Student Nursing

ABOUT THE SERIES EDITORS

DR MOOI STANDING is an Independent Nursing Consultant (UK and International) and is responsible for the core knowledge, adult nursing and personal and professional learning skills titles. She is an experienced NMC Quality Assurance Reviewer of educational programmes and Professional Regulator Panellist on the NMC Practice Committee. Mooi is also Board member of Special Olympics Malaysia, enabling people with intellectual disabilities to participate in sports and athletics nationally and internationally.

DR SANDRA WALKER is a Clinical Academic in Mental Health working between Southern Health Trust and the University of Southampton and responsible for the mental health nursing titles. She is a Qualified Mental Health Nurse with a wide range of clinical experience spanning more than 25 years.

BESTSELLING TEXTBOOKS

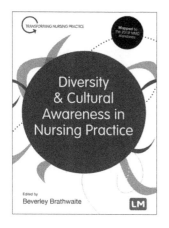

Diversity & Cultural Awareness in Nursing Practice

Edited by Beverley Brathwaite

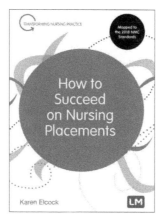

How to Succeed on Nursing Placements

Karen Elcock

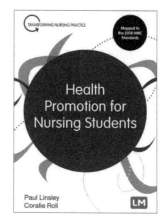

Health Promotion for Nursing Students

Paul Linsley
Coralie Roll

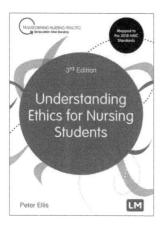

3rd Edition

Understanding Ethics for Nursing Students

Peter Ellis

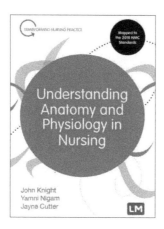

Understanding Anatomy and Physiology in Nursing

John Knight
Yamni Nigam
Jayne Cutter

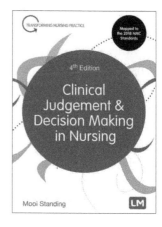

4th Edition

Clinical Judgement & Decision Making in Nursing

Mooi Standing

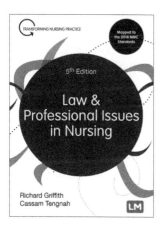

5th Edition

Law & Professional Issues in Nursing

Richard Griffith
Cassam Tengnah

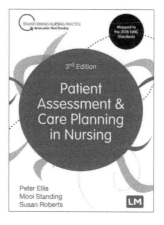

3rd Edition

Patient Assessment & Care Planning in Nursing

Peter Ellis
Mooi Standing
Susan Roberts

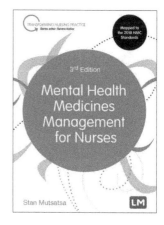

3rd Edition

Mental Health Medicines Management for Nurses

Stan Mutsatsa

You can find a full list of textbooks in the *Transforming Nursing Practice* series at
https://uk.sagepub.com

Foreword

Critical Thinking and Writing in Nursing facilitates the development of essential personal and professional learning skills by carefully guiding readers in how to process information and then articulate what they have learned. Readers' personal development is facilitated in acquiring, understanding and demonstrating critical thinking, reflecting and scholarly writing skills. This goes hand in hand with their professional development as they are given useful tips on how to make best use of the wide variety of learning situations that they experience, as well as how to apply critical thinking skills in formal academic and practical assessments. Readers are encouraged to engage with lots of interesting and challenging activities that combine and progressively stretch their personal and professional learning skills in reflecting and thinking critically. The book utilises the experience of four nursing students during their nursing programme as a useful device to illustrate different perspectives and learning styles in acquiring and applying critical thinking skills. This offers a helpful reference point for readers to gauge their own development in this respect while broadening their appreciation and understanding of others' unique viewpoints. The needs of registered nurses are accommodated by relating critical thinking and reflection to revalidation requirements. This is nicely illustrated by incorporating an ongoing case study of a registered nurse to compare and contrast with the four nursing students. Innovative frameworks are provided to help readers identify and understand different levels of reflection and critical thinking, as well as how they are applied in nursing and healthcare. This is very helpful for nursing students to understand what is expected of them at different stages of their programme, as well as how they might achieve this. The author also explains how critical thinking and reflection enables nurses (or nursing associates) to fulfil their professional duties in *The Code* (NMC, 2018a) and meet the Standards of Proficiency for Registered Nurses (NMC, 2018b) – for example, showing how critical thinking skills are vital in enhancing patient care by relating the theory of person-centred, safe, effective, evidence-based nursing interventions to practice.

In the fifth edition of this highly regarded book, the author has incorporated changes that take account of new developments and feedback, as well as his continued commitment to make a complex topic understandable and helpful to readers. Significant revisions have been made, including a new chapter, 'Writing the clinical case study', which links theory to practice by demonstrating how readers can apply critical thinking skills to evaluate the care they have provided or witnessed. There are also useful additional learning tools included that help readers to recognise and utilise different kinds of information and emotional intelligence, within a template of critical thinking, which enhances effective person-centred care. I wholeheartedly recommend this excellent book to all nursing students, registered nurses, practice supervisors/assessors and nurse educators.

Dr Mooi Standing
Series Editor

Acknowledgements

The first edition of this book began as a collaborative venture between myself and Dr Anne Harrington. We agreed that nursing students needed help to develop as critical thinkers, using their learning and experience to best effect. I would like to thank Anne for her work on the previous editions and for sharing my enthusiasm to help students make a success of their courses. This book would not have been possible, however, without the further contributions of Stewart, Fatima, Raymet, Gina and Sue, who very generously agreed to explore critical thinking and reflection with us through their own work. The book certainly would not have made it to the printed and e-learning pages without the support and very constructive feedback of critical readers, series editor Dr Mooi Standing and the editorial team at SAGE.

About the author

Bob Price is a healthcare education and training consultant. Formerly, he was Director, Postgraduate Awards in Advancing Healthcare Practice at the Open University. A passionate educator, he has assisted students at every level, from pre-registration programmes of study up to and including PhD. Bob's doctoral thesis was on the negotiation of learning and strategies used by students and tutors to develop scholarly and professional forms of expression. He is an editorial advisor to a range of healthcare journals, advising editors on teaching texts and student learning needs.

Introduction

The ability to think critically, to reflect upon experience and then to write about such matters in a clear fashion is central to your success, both while studying a programme of nursing studies and later when demonstrating your readiness to revalidate as a registered nurse (NMC, 2019). *The Code* (NMC, 2018a) requires nurses to attend safely, sensitively, effectively, imaginatively and efficiently to patient care, and this is underpinned by both critical thinking and reflection. This book is designed to assist you with this process: the making sense of that which is read, taught or encountered; the translation of information into learning; and the representation of learning in coursework, or as information required by the NMC (revalidation).

The book has a further purpose, however – one that is very personal. This relates to helping you to think in ways that help you to endure within nursing. Healthcare practice is full of challenges and possibilities. While we work within a code of practice and with clinical guidelines and protocols, there are many different ways to care for patients. There are often difficulties in negotiating the right care with patients and their families. There are equally challenges associated with allocating scant resources and prioritising care when demands compete for your time. While much is taught to you, and much is recommended, you will still have to deliberate on what is practicable, ethical and professional in care delivery. What is acceptable to the patient (informed consent), what is recommended as ideal (professional philosophy) and what is practicable (health service economics) are not always the same. Addressing the many competing demands about what you should do is stressful. For that reason, this book is also about judging the practical utility of information, theories and arguments. Success in your career may sometimes depend upon the skill you have in navigating the practical as well as the desirable.

Nursing presents us with a flood of information – gleaned from lectures, demonstrations, seminars and workshops, programmes of reading, electronic forum discussions, study days and conferences, and what you discover through clinical practice. Within higher education today, greater emphasis is placed upon discovery and collaborative learning – you 'read for a degree'. Many enquiries involve library- or practice-based, work augmented by lectures and tutorials. If past education involved more teaching and listening, you will find now that you have to be rather more proactive and inquisitive in your approach. Processing information in the right way takes time and benefits from wise counsel. As a student, you will naturally wish to liaise closely with your tutors as part of this work. If you are already a registered nurse, then a manager, clinical leader or more experienced colleague is often a good source of counsel. As you think about what you have learned and prepare for coursework assessment, this book should prove valuable.

Who is this book for?

This book has been written for two audiences: students completing nursing courses (basic and post-basic levels) and registered nurses who are charged with demonstrating their continued learning and enquiry as part of the revalidation process (NMC, 2019). While the requirements of critical thinking and reflection may vary (e.g. associated with the level of course studied), the processes remain much the same. The nurse has to process that which is discovered, interpreting and sorting it before care decisions can be made.

Because the book starts with the basics, it is designed to reassure and support those of you who may not have studied for some time. I begin with the assumption that critical thinking, reflecting and writing are three of the craft skills of nursing.

Much of what is best in nursing is defined by the way in which we deliver care as much as by what is provided. For this reason, reading this book will start you on a journey where you discover how best to use your experience in the service of others. This is a process that draws heavily upon making sense of practice, exploring what you believe is best within nursing care, and planning future development that helps you to express your thinking more effectively.

Critical thinking and reflecting

One of the earliest discoveries made by student nurses is how often the word 'critical' appears in their work. In the clinical context, the word carries connotations of risk and the need for urgent intervention (e.g. 'a patient is critically ill') (Odell, 2015). Used in this sense, the nurse quickly realises the need for precision and judgement, the requirement to do the right thing, in the right way and at the right time. In the academic context, 'critical' takes on several different meanings (Merisier et al., 2018). You are asked to 'critically discuss', 'critically evaluate' and 'critically explore' a subject, and it slowly becomes apparent that to be critical involves different things, depending on the teaching or assessment involved. For example, to be critical in this context might mean to discriminate between what is right and wrong, defensible and indefensible. Asking the right questions of information or a clinical situation is important. If you are preparing a reflective piece of writing, then 'critical' often involves being introspective, examining afresh your beliefs, values and motives.

In this book, I use the term 'critical thinking' in a precise way. It describes the process by which we develop powers of analysis and investigation, as well as enhancing our ability to discriminate what is relevant and to discern what might prove most helpful. Critical thinking may have to work in situations where there is no absolute truth, no perfect answers, only better ones. Much as we might yearn for certainty, there are times in healthcare when none can be promised.

Critical thinking involves judgement, and nurses are frequently assessed on their decision-making skills (Kavanagh and Szweda, 2017). A competent nurse is one who selects the relevant information to plan a course of action and then judges what is best to do in a given circumstance (Casey et al., 2017). We are best placed to meet registration standards and to improve care where we have the capacity to reason what is not yet understood and what will enable us to be more imaginative, sensitive, respectful, and efficient and effective in what we do.

While 'critical' is sometimes encountered in a more destructive form within practice (e.g. where practitioners belittle others' shortfalls), this is not the sense in which we will use it here. Indeed, I suggest that the individual who criticises without consideration of what is learned through the experience is demonstrating neither scholarship nor professionalism.

It is likely that you have already engaged in reflection as part of previous studies. For example, at school, you perhaps judged which subjects to take to examination based on your past comfort with them in class. However, in nursing, reflection has a very important and specific role. It is strongly associated with the development of empathy (i.e. the understanding of and respect for the circumstances of others) (McKinnon, 2018). Nurses need to be emotionally intelligent, as well as anticipating how illness, treatment and care might seem to patients and how different courses of action might seem to professional colleagues. Without adequate empathy, there is a significant risk that patients may be neglected. Because nurses are asked to use their experience and their insights as part of nursing care, reflection takes on a special meaning. While at least some of your teaching in college starts with concepts or theories that describe the world of healthcare, much of what you learn through practice starts from episodes of care that are much more ambiguous. We have to make sense of what is going on. Evidence alone will not secure the healthcare improvements that nurses and others strive for. Not surprisingly, then, both critical thinking and reflection are centre stage within this book. Critical thinking engages our reasoning as we ponder theories, evidence, arguments and debates, while reflection does the same as we contemplate experience.

How this book is set out

This book is set out in three parts. You will certainly benefit from reading it cover to cover, but it will also serve you when you wish to 'dip into' particular chapters later. Part 1 consists of three chapters that introduce you in an accessible way to the key concepts which feature in this book: critical thinking, reflecting, and scholarly writing. Securing a basic idea about what these concepts are all about will help you to make a great deal more sense of what is asked of you within the nursing syllabus. Within Part 1, I introduce you to different levels of critical thinking and reflection, something that you will need to understand in order to pass module assessments.

Part 2 concerns the use of reasoning and reflection within different contexts. It will help you to understand what is involved in getting the most from a variety of learning opportunities, including lectures, demonstrations, seminars, workshops and clinical placements. Much of what I write about here relating to learning in university contexts applies equally well to the registered nurse preparing for revalidation. Conferences and study days, for example, are often arranged as a series of lectures and smaller 'breakout' group discussions.

As you study Part 2, it is important to remember that there is usually method in what could seem a perverse curriculum. You are asked to engage in different learning activities for a reason, and this includes building confidence in your own enquiries. It is not the teacher's objective to drill you in a set way of thinking. Rather, they hope to acquaint you with different approaches to enquiry and understanding. Sometimes teaching precedes a programme of library enquiry. You are assisted in deducing things, such as whether a theory holds good in all circumstances. Sometimes you are tasked with individual or group enquiries in order to build a theory of your own (inductive learning). The organisation of studies within a module will have a specific purpose, although they may seem discomfiting or obtuse at times! Your course is likely to require very active learning; it will not be sufficient to sit, wait and take notes.

If Part 2 is about the process of learning, then Part 3 is about the process of expressing what you have learned. This part opens with a chapter on evaluating evidence. During your nursing career, you will have access to a wide range of evidence of varying quality, so it is vital that you can reason to best effect here. We assist you with the matter of writing different sorts of essays (analytical and reflective) and building a portfolio that helps you to demonstrate your progress. While there are many forms that assessment can take in nursing courses, the principles of analytical and reflective writing remain firm. In this part, we spend some time illustrating how you can demonstrate the different levels of critical thinking that may be required at different stages of your course. Part 3 also includes a new chapter on writing clinical case studies, something that will be important when justifying the planning of patient support over a series of care episodes. The clinical case study helps you to link reflective practice skills and critical analysis of evidence together.

Learning features

Throughout the book, you will find activities that will help you to make sense of and learn about the material presented.

Some of the activities ask you to *reflect* on aspects of practice. Other activities ask you to *think critically* about a topic in order to challenge received wisdom. You may be asked to *research a topic and find appropriate information and evidence*, as well as to be able to *make decisions* using that evidence.

All of the activities require you to take a break from reading the text, think through the issues presented, and carry out some independent study, possibly using the internet. You might want to think about completing the activities as part of your portfolio.

NMC Standards of Proficiency for Registered Nurses

In 2018, the UK's NMC published its Standards of Proficiency for Registered Nurses (NMC, 2018b), describing what registered nurses must be able to demonstrate at the conclusion of their nurse education. Relevant standards are detailed at the start of each chapter in this book.

Supporting the NMC code of professional practice

In addition to the above standards, this book works closely with the NMC code of professional practice (*The Code*).

The Code (NMC, 2018a) describes four areas of professional responsibility:

- prioritise people;
- practise effectively;
- preserve safety;
- promote professionalism and trust.

Prioritise people

Nurses are required to attend quickly, considerately, respectfully and compassionately to other people, both the service users within healthcare and their colleagues in practice. Nurses must be able to analyse others' likely needs and concerns, as well as respecting their confidentiality and individuality while doing so. It is important for nurses to listen to the experience of patients and what they have to relate about their expectations of care.

If you are to prioritise people successfully, it is vital that you learn to think critically about their situation and needs. A patient may not know all of their concerns, needs and risks immediately, so you will have to be adept at identifying potential problems. Learning about how best to ask questions, as well as evaluating the information that you secure from them, is a vital part of planning individualised care. Chapter 1 teaches you about critical thinking and Chapter 6 helps you to build confidence in thinking in a more critical way when you learn in the practice setting. Chapter 2 introduces you to reflection as a process. Much of what you learn about delivering care in an individualised way comes from learning directly with and from patients.

Practise effectively

It is not enough that nurses are respectful and considerate towards patients; they must be effective as well. Healthcare resources, be they medicines, materials or the nurse's time, are scarce resources and must be used to best effect. To work effectively, *The Code* requires that nurses make the best possible use of evidence, communicate clearly, work cooperatively, and share their skills and expertise with others.

Critical thinking (Chapter 1) is important in efficient and effective practice. What will work best, and why? What is the best order in which to do things? Why might it be better to act in one way than another? Chapter 8 helps you to better understand evidence that stems from research, clinical audit and clinical case studies. Although evidence may recommend a particular course of action, it may not seem the best or most desirable course of action to the patient, so reflection (Chapter 2) is important here as well. A nurse might need to 'sell' the benefits of a recommended course of action to a patient.

Preserve safety

Nurses have the potential to cause considerable harm and to do great good. With this in mind, *The Code* requires that nurses work within the limits of their competence, as well as within the protocols and policies established by healthcare organisations. They must be prepared to raise concerns where patients seem at risk and to intervene in emergencies where they have the requisite competence to do so. Nurses must be prepared to acknowledge mistakes or errors, as well as acting quickly and collaboratively to mitigate these where possible.

Judging exactly what you know, as well as how confident this might make you feel, is important. What you read about in Chapter 1 (critical thinking) and Chapter 2 (reflection), as well as what you learn in Chapter 3 (scholarly writing), will prompt you to examine again what supports your decision-making. Safety often relies upon judging when not to act, when it is better to consult or refer, and this in turn relies upon a willingness to examine why something seems like a good idea. Critical thinking, reflection and case-making, then, are important in making better and safer decisions.

Promote professionalism and trust

The Code reminds nurses of their professional responsibility to uphold the reputation of the profession, as well as their own status as a nurse. To this end, they must act without favour and not accept loans or gifts that might otherwise influence their professional judgement or the reputation of the profession. They must respond promptly and considerately to complaints, as well as exercising leadership as part of their work to promote the well-being of patients and excellence in care standards. Registered nurses are expected to carry on learning, refining and improving their professional skills, and mastering new knowledge or approaches to care that reflect what evidence has taught.

Being ready to examine complaints honestly, as well as confronting suspect practice, relies upon our readiness to judge evidence and explain our reasoning. What is excellent? What is suspect? What could lead to harm or difficulty for the patient? We will need to think objectively and critically (Chapter 1), as well as reflecting on events, even though this causes us to revisit our own values and beliefs (Chapter 2). Chapter 12 introduces you to the benefits of building and maintaining a professional portfolio.

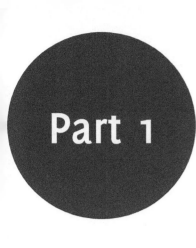

Part 1   Understanding thinking, reflecting and writing

Chapter 1 Critical thinking

NMC Standards of Proficiency for Registered Nurses

This chapter will address the following platforms and proficiencies:

Platform 1: Being an accountable professional

At the point of registration, the registered nurse will be able to:

1.8 Demonstrate the knowledge, skills and ability to think critically when applying evidence and drawing on experience to make evidence informed decisions in all situations.

1.9 Understand the need to base all decisions regarding care and interventions on people's needs and preferences, recognising and addressing any personal and external factors that may unduly influence their decisions.

1.18 Demonstrate the knowledge and confidence to contribute effectively and proactively in an interdisciplinary team.

Platform 3: Assessing needs and planning care

At the point of registration, the registered nurse will be able to:

3.5 Demonstrate the ability to accurately process all information gathered during the assessment process to identify needs for individualised nursing care and develop person-centred evidence-based plans for nursing interventions with agreed goals.

3.7 Understand and apply the principles and processes for making reasonable adjustments.

Platform 5: Leading and managing nursing care and working in teams

At the point of registration, the registered nurse will be able to:

5.1 Understand the principles of effective leadership, management, group and organisational dynamics and culture and apply these to team working and decision-making.

Chapter aims

....

After reading this chapter, you will be able to:

- define critical thinking in your own practical terms, using illustrations as necessary;
- discuss why this skill is important in nursing;
- summarise different aptitudes associated with critical thinking;
- indicate your level of confidence associated with each of the aptitudes of critical thinking;
- describe what constitutes more sophisticated forms of critical thinking.

Introduction

Shortly, we will begin exploring critical thinking as a key nursing skill, one that is essential for your studies. Before I do that, however, let us set this skill in context. Your career in nursing has never been more dependent upon the ability to reason in a critical way. Critical thinking is essential for your personal well-being and your sense of purposeful work. Here are three contexts that highlight this:

1. The knowledge that we use to nurse today is considerably greater than it ever was before, and it comprises a mass of sometimes contradictory, incomplete or contentious information (Rodgers et al., 2018). We have much greater access to information of varying quality. This has profound implications when patients ask you for advice, evaluate what you do, and explore their own hopes for healthcare. If we do not know how to evaluate complex information, to conceptualise to best effect, then we will struggle to be effective, compassionate and imaginative carers.

2. Our knowledge operates where there remains a gulf between what could be done and what philosophers and leaders believe should be done (Salifu et al., 2019). Just as the demands of health consumers have increased, so have the aspirations of nursing as a profession. We hope to care better, and this has usually focused upon more bespoke care. What could and should be done, however, often conflict during nursing shifts. Your skills and expertise have to work in real time in settings where time and material resources are at a premium. You cannot promise to deliver everything that everyone desires, so you must make difficult decisions about what you offer to stakeholders such as patients and relatives. Those decisions involve the strategic use of information. This prompts new questions: How utilisable is nursing knowledge? Can I make these ideas work? Just how important such questions are becomes apparent when you consider stress in nursing. Our ability to sustain a lifelong career in nursing depends, in part, on juggling a large number

of expectations, feeling that we have made a realistic and meaningful contribution (Fasbender et al., 2018).

3. Nursing knowledge today operates within the context of shifting roles and responsibilities (Schober, 2019). What we do today is very different to what nurses did 20 years ago. In many areas, this means that practice is extended and nurses do work that doctors did previously. But it may also mean that sometimes nurses focus on much more discreet areas of care. For example, a nurse might act as a counsellor with a specialist clientele. Once upon a time, nurses talked about 'basic nursing care', but today we might struggle to agree what 'basic' means. In a world of shifting roles, it becomes challenging to decide how far your responsibilities extend. You will need critical thinking to feel that you have a clear purpose and a consistent career direction to follow.

Activity 1.1   Reflection

Reflect now upon some of the media stories that you have watched or read about concerning the health services and nursing. Do these seem to emphasise a need for critical thinking? For example, if care is criticised as inadequate, does an understanding of knowledge in use help us to evaluate that which is observed? Because media stories may vary widely and change over time, I have not offered further thoughts at the chapter end. What I do suggest, however, is that critical thinking is increasingly important to the ways in which nursing care is both experienced and represented. What nursing is, how it is judged, is often understood in terms of care explained.

Critical thinking

We have been involved in reasoning throughout our lives. However, many of the past decisions that we have made have been managed in a tacit way (i.e. without great analysis). To be successful nurses, though, we need to practise the skill of critical thinking in a more conscious manner (Standing, 2020).

Critical thinking can be described as having two foci. The first entails the careful scrutiny of phenomena, causes, consequences, correlations and contexts. These are **empirical** things, facts, statistics, tests and results. This involves the exercise of what has been called **cognitive intelligence** (Jenicek, 2018). When you assess a wound, for example, you examine the extent and depth of the wound, whether it is infected, and whether in the light of treatment it is improving. The assessment is dispassionate and measured. But in nursing, critical thinking also involves an understanding of how we and others feel (e.g. what it involves to be ill). This is **emotional intelligence** (Mangubat, 2017). Nurses need to exercise emotional intelligence in order to deliver care sensitively.

What, then, do we mean by critical thinking? As Lovatt (2014) notes, a definition is difficult to pin down, and each represents something of a compromise. However, it seems important to share with you my definition. For me, critical thinking is:

> *A process where different information is gathered, sifted, synthesised and evaluated in order to understand a subject or issue. Critical thinking engages our intellect (the ability to discriminate, challenge and argue), but it might engage our emotions too. To think critically, we need to take account of values, beliefs and attitudes that shape our perceptions. Critical thinking, then, is that which enables the nurse to function as a knowledgeable practitioner – someone who selects, combines, judges and uses information in order to proceed in a professional manner. Critical thinking is vital if we are to act strategically and to convey our care and compassion for others.*

Critical thinking and learning

To help you explore further, I now introduce you to four student nurses and one staff nurse. Stewart, Fatima, Raymet and Gina are students, while Sue is a staff nurse on a busy hospital ward. Sue's interest is in the use of critical thinking to prepare for revalidation (NMC, 2019), but she remembers what study was like. We will return to our case study nurses periodically throughout the book.

Our case study nurses meet up to discuss some of the challenges of completing a nursing course. While their studies are interesting, they all acknowledge that learning can be difficult because of the critical thinking required.

Activity 1.2   Reflection

Look now at the accounts in the box below of critical thinking challenges reported by our group.

- Have you encountered similar concerns?
- Why do you think that making connections between teaching and practice (Stewart), managing uncertainty (Fatima), dealing with large volumes of information (Raymet), and knowing what to do and how to do it (Gina) tells us about how nurses have to think?

As this answer is based on your own observation, there is no outline answer at the end of the chapter.

Case study: Five critical thinking challenges

Stewart:	'I've realised not only that there is important theory to grasp, but that it isn't always simple to use in practice. Not everything in theory seems open to use. Some of it has to be adjusted before you can use it. Maybe some of it is just nice to know?'
Fatima:	'For me, it's the uncertainty. I long for a right answer, something that I know is just correct, and a lot of what we're learning about – for instance, ethics – isn't so clear-cut.'
Raymet:	'I agree! But have you noticed just how much information there is? It's like they fill up your kitbag with everything you could ever want and then leave you to decide when to pull it out. The sheer volume is worrying.'
Gina:	'I wouldn't disagree with any of those points. But have you noticed how important it is to understand processes as well as purposes? You quickly learn what you should do, but how to do it is something more complex. It's that which I find myself admiring nurses for.'
Sue (registered nurse):	'Goodness, I remember those anxieties! The learning I do now for professional update is less structured than before. I have to decide what I wish to know, to improve upon, and then to judge the best ways to meet my needs. That means sometimes confronting care that I didn't get right. It means being candid with myself about the need to improve what I do.'

You may already be empathising with these five colleagues, each of whom captures something about critical thinking in nursing. Nursing practice relies heavily on the skills of the nurse, and central among these is the ability to reason. Skills are made up of a series of component parts, and it is the way in which these are combined and used that determines how skilful the practice seems (Gobet, 2005; Gobet and Chassy, 2008; Sala and Gobet, 2017) (see Figure 1.1). While the circumstances under which critical thinking must be exercised may change (e.g. an emergency versus palliative care), expert practitioners are still able to combine the components of critical thinking in ways which serve well (Sala and Gobet, 2017). This is because the ways of thinking in different situations (templates) are repeatedly tested by the nurse.

In the case study above, Stewart refers to the first of these components. Stewart worries about the application of theory. If we are going to deliver good nursing care, we have to know how to combine and apply information. But information does not fit everywhere. So, for example, a series of seminars on grief might have value with dying patients or those who have lost a bodily function, but wider application may be limited (it has limited **utility**). Not all information gleaned can be immediately used, nor is it universally taught for use in practice. Sometimes we learn things to appreciate how nursing has evolved. That said, however, we are usually faced with a challenge. We have to be able to declare certain things (as true, sound, proven and/or relevant) if we are to develop the confidence to proceed. Without that, we feel paralysed when facing clinical situations. What we need, then, is knowledge that has a frequent fit with clinical demands. It is not unreasonable to discuss the best fit use of information with your tutor. How abstract is the theory? Does it recognise the differences between patients, their histories and cultural backgrounds, for example?

Activity 1.3   Reflection

Try now to think of something within nursing that you must be able to assert confidently which also has utility (i.e. it is workable) in your chosen area of recent practice.

An outline answer is given at the end of this chapter.

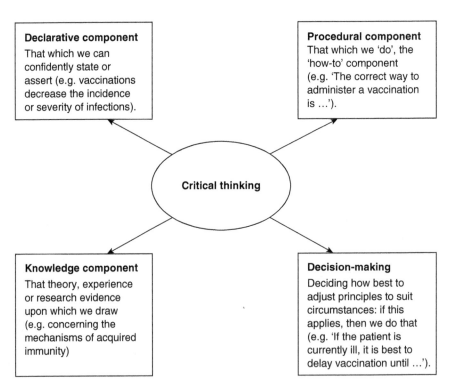

Declarative component
That which we can confidently state or assert (e.g. vaccinations decrease the incidence or severity of infections).

Procedural component
That which we 'do', the 'how-to' component (e.g. 'The correct way to administer a vaccination is ...').

Critical thinking

Knowledge component
That theory, experience or research evidence upon which we draw (e.g. concerning the mechanisms of acquired immunity)

Decision-making
Deciding how best to adjust principles to suit circumstances: if this applies, then we do that (e.g. 'If the patient is currently ill, it is best to delay vaccination until ...').

Figure 1.1   Critical thinking components of nursing skill

Fatima refers to a second important component of critical thinking: *decision-making.* There is often no 'one-size-fits-all' solution. Fatima is keenly aware that nurses have to deal with uncertainty, sometimes waiting to gather more information before making a decision. Living with such uncertainty, especially in clinical practice, is what can seem stressful for nurses. They have to learn to read developing situations and weigh the merits of different courses of action.

Raymet is worried about how best to artfully select and combine information to make excellent decisions. Established nurses seem to do it easily, explaining that they use 'nous', but Raymet is unsure what that is. The practice supervisors she has met describe it as a mix of thinking, remembering (from **experience**) and reading (how patients and relatives respond). We can only reason effectively if we have amassed a sufficient quantity of high-quality knowledge that makes sense in the context of care (Ellis, 2019). Nurses have to speculate how different bits of information might fit together to imagine how a plan of action might seem to patients. They have to use both cognitive and emotional intelligence.

Activity 1.4   Reflection

Identify now one example of a difficult decision that you know about from clinical practice, or one that was debated in class. Was the decision of the either/or kind or was it more complicated, with multiple options and the merit of each dependent on factors such as patient preference?

Next jot down what you understand the term 'nous' to mean.

An outline answer is given at the end of this chapter.

Both Gina and Sue refer to the *process* part of the skill. Reasoning is not only concerned with deciding what knowledge is appropriate, determining what is true, safe or effective, and making judicious decisions; it is also concerned with how you plan your work. When a nurse gives an injection, they determine the right order in which to proceed. For example, the nurse forewarns the patient about the planned injection, secures consent, and then ensures a private environment to help to protect the patient's dignity. Sue reflects on the process of further enquiry, first by confronting deficits in your practice, accepting a need to learn more, and then deciding how best to go about that. Planning the right sequence of work is important, whether completing a clinical procedure or planning update enquiries.

Activity 1.5   Critical thinking

Explore now with a chosen colleague an activity from your recent learning to determine the different ways in which reasoning has had to work (deciding what you can claim, making decisions, reviewing knowledge and deciding on process). Next compare notes with your colleague on which of the skill components seemed toughest, and why.

Because this activity focuses on your chosen learning activity, no additional remarks are added at the end of the chapter.

In my experience, it is often the **declarative critical thinking** component of a skill that seems hardest to students. There is sometimes no single 'right' answer, but there are better answers. To ascertain those, discussion and consultation with others is so important. That is why nursing courses build in so much discussion time and why you are asked to 'think aloud'. Qualified nurses confront the declarative skills component problem by conferring with colleagues and sometimes collaborating on case conferences. It is professionally important that nurses acknowledge what they are unsure about and are candid about any dilemmas which they face (NMC, 2018a).

No matter what part of the course you are studying, you will be engaged in critical thinking, combining and recombining the different components of nursing skills so that you can proceed in ways which seem professional. Nursing practice has to be reasoned, and the actions of the nurse reasonable. Indeed, in a court of law, judgements about whether a nurse's actions are negligent are based upon what a reasonable practitioner would do (Baylis, 2015). What the case study nurses will learn throughout their course is designed to enable them to work more safely, strategically, effectively (achieving required outcomes) and efficiently (using resources wisely).

Building templates

You might wonder, what next? Once we appreciate that critical thinking involves these different skill components, what follows on from that? The brief answer is that you start to develop some **templates** to make better sense of what you have discovered, what you have been taught, and what you might then do. This process is called **conceptualisation** – clustering information together to make useful wholes. A list of concepts that nurses regularly use might include pain, recovery, rehabilitation, support and effective listening. When the concepts include practical actions, responses to needs or concerns, we call them templates. 'Template' sounds like a technical term, but it simply means a working explanation of what we encounter and how we can best respond. Human beings develop templates from childhood (Gold et al., 2016). For example, babies learn very quickly to make distinctions between what is threatening and what is comforting. A smile represents friendliness and a glare represents threat. As you get older, you develop strategies to respond to friendliness and threat – you have been building templates for a good many years.

In nursing, though, the building of templates has to be rather more conscious. Much of your teaching is designed to help you to do that. The very best practice supervisors are able to explain how they assess practice situations – they share their working templates. I asked Sue (our case study registered nurse) to help with this using an example of a template that she uses nearly every day of her working life. She chose anxiety. Patients and their families frequently exhibit anxiety, and the nurse needs a working template to deal with it. Here is what she told me:

> *Anxiety is something you recognise as a pattern. Certain things go together again and again, and that enables you to predict what might cause anxiety and how it will emerge.*

When you anticipate it well and move to reassure the patient, they appreciate your care. So, for anxiety, the pattern includes things like sudden change, a lack of or too much information, words and terms that seem very technical, and doubts about their ability to control what happens next. That is the pattern of anxiety. You counter anxiety using different tools – reassurance, yes, but giving patients room to express their fears as well. So, if you keep checking your solutions against anxiety, you develop a working template. It's something you can use while staying ready to think again if something new pops up.

Your course is designed to help you to develop working templates that will help you to practise nursing. That is why you are taught theory, why you share seminars (exploring what works together, what fits), and why it is good to ask practice supervisors about how they read clinical situations. When we think critically, we hope to recognise patterns of information, those that represent something important to us (e.g. risk, rehabilitation, relapse, cancer, depression, compassion).

To build these templates, though, we are going to have to engage in some important work that connects reasoning to study.

Making critical thinking work for you

I asked the case study nurses to tell me what seemed to count as critical thinking in their nursing course, what seemed to be especially valued. I wanted to know what they thought was welcomed by tutors. What they told me is shown in Table 1.1.

Student	Aptitude	The student said …
Stewart	Asking questions	'If you don't ask questions, then you simply accept others' explanations, and that could be wrong. You have to be respectfully inquisitive.'
Fatima	Discriminating	'I find that you need to show how you reach conclusions, weighing up information. You have to show that you've thought about what is relevant.'
Raymet	Making arguments	'I don't think you can just hide behind what others have claimed. You have to explain what you think and take a considered stance.'
Gina	Interpreting and speculating	'I think that you show why you think something is significant, so you explain why you focus on it. But it is also important to say when you are speculating what could be the case. Don't be arrogant.'

Table 1.1   Critical thinking aptitudes

Asking questions

Asking questions is certainly important, but individuals vary in their levels of confidence. Perhaps you worry that asking questions suggests an uncomfortable level of ignorance. Asking questions, though, especially when working with professional colleagues, is at the heart of healthcare. For example, questions are frequently used to clarify the best care options, and at best these involve patients being involved in decisions. Sometimes a seemingly naive question is the one that transforms everyone's understanding of a clinical situation. You may hear practice supervisors rehearsing questions aloud as an aid to planning care: 'If I want to teach Mrs Jones about her insulin therapy, what does she need to understand in order to keep her safe and help her to master injection-giving?'

You can improve your question-asking by:

- deciding exactly what you need to know – this will help you to be precise as regards what you ask about;
- formulating your question in a way that establishes your focus of interest – it is better, for instance, to link a question about patient experience to a contextual concern, such as preoperative anxiety;
- jotting down your question before you ask it – this will help you to explain what you wish to understand.

Discriminating

There comes a stage where we have to discriminate between what is relevant and what is irrelevant, as well as what is true and what is false. Discrimination involves weighing up information and determining what enables us to make arguments that might be supported by others. One example of discrimination in action is where a nurse searches for evidence to support a given practice. The nurse reasons that the information supplied through research studies is superior to that derived from anecdotal evidence, at least where the design of research has been rigorous. If you are judging the claims made by others, one way of showing discrimination is to ponder the circumstances or conditions under which an argument might be false. 'Under what conditions might it be unsafe for the patient to remain at home to receive care?' is an example of a question that might be used.

A part of discrimination involves judging what is operable, what can work in practice. Is theory always operable? Person-centred care, for example, is a theory that has significant appeal for nurses (myself included), but it does make significant demands on patients as partners. The extent that we can demonstrate it may depend on the patient's readiness to collaborate, as well as the nurse's skill (Price, 2019a)

Showing appropriate discrimination in your reasoning will be important in your written work. You will need to demonstrate that you have considered possible explanations of what you have read, as well as determining what you need to consider before you elect a particular course of action. In Part 3, we discuss different levels of critical thinking in your writing, and one of the markers of higher-level critical thinking is that not only can you identify what must be discriminated between (the competing explanations), but you can also reason why one explanation seems better than another. Where writing shows little or no recognition of competing explanations, it might be described as uncritical or even opinionated.

Making arguments

Arguments are formulated about a variety of things: what should be done next, what this literature suggests, and what constitutes compassionate care. Arguments are necessary, as they explain the basis of nursing in action and why we are working to the goals that we have. An argument is made up of a case (what we believe is true) and **premises** (the things that support the case) (Chatfield, 2018; Price, 2019b). Both the case and the constituent premises may be supported by research evidence, audit and experience. So, for example, we might make an argument about patient anxiety and how it interferes with collaborative care planning: 'Collaborative care planning is made more difficult with anxious patients (the case) because patients have a limited command of relevant information and they feel less powerful than clinicians (two supporting premises).' Notice the importance of the word 'because'. If we do not include what follows after it, we only present an opinion. We can only evaluate the argument if we understand on what basis the case is presented.

Classically, an argument such as this is judged with regard to whether the premises and the case fit well together. Are the premises sufficient to support the case? But we might also consider whether the argument seems complete. There may be other factors that affect collaborative care planning (e.g. clinicians' willingness to consult with patients).

In nursing, the rationale for an argument may be based on evidence, but it might also be based on **moral justice** (Grace, 2017). Some arguments are made on ethical grounds regarding what *should* be done. In clinical practice, a wide variety of factors impinge upon arguments made, including those relating to patient rights and anticipated outcomes. A good way to strengthen your arguments within a debate is to show that you have carefully considered alternative arguments, namely other ways to see the situation. You then reject weaker arguments by offering a rationale for why they are not valid (the premises do not support the case), relevant or realistic, given the context in which care is delivered.

Activity 1.6 Collaborative practice

Have a go now formulating an argument for your colleagues to interrogate. Remember that the argument needs a case (that which you claim) and premises that support it. Typically, the case is presented first, and then after 'because' come the underpinning premises. Did your colleagues support your argument or did they counter it? If it seemed weak, what do you think

(Continued)

(Continued)

the problem was? An unclear case, weak premises, the wrong premises? Remember that your coursework will often need to include arguments, so what you test out here could be especially valuable.

As this answer is based on your own observation, there is no outline answer at the end of the chapter.

Interpreting and speculating

Interpreting involves making sense of that which is encountered. A variety of stimuli are received by the nurse (e.g. auditory and visual information) and these are converted into perceptions (impressions) when the nurse combines this information with past experiences (memories). Successful interpretation then relies upon being alert to all of the possible information, and then understanding how this can be combined to determine what is happening (Cooper and Frain, 2016). Sometimes conflicting information will be encountered that makes it harder for the nurse to decide what the information signals (e.g. risk, improvement, deterioration, sepsis, a new stage of illness). Nevertheless, interpreting is an important skill element because it links enquiry to the formulation of the templates that you have already read about. Eventually, enough information might amass, tested against research and experience, for the nurse to say that there is a clear pattern which represents patient anxiety. This is important, and we must act in these ways if patients are not to suffer unduly.

While searching for such patterns is most readily related to clinical demands, it is also important in your campus studies. A literature search may, for instance, suggest that recurring themes arise on your chosen topic. Imagine that you were investigating disfigurement and its effect on patient well-being. If the literature repeatedly threw up the importance of injury context (e.g. an acid attack) for the degree of distress that a disfigurement causes, it would be reasonable to highlight that in your analysis. We search for patterns of information to help determine where we enquire next and how we might respond.

I have left **speculation** until last, and consider it extremely important. Successful nursing relies in large part on nurses 'thinking outside the box', daring to consider options or solutions that are unfamiliar. Creativity and imagination therefore form a valuable part of critical thinking, one that can help nurses to improve the lot of patients.

Sue talks about a nurse that she admired:

One specialist nurse I knew pulled all of the information together about teaching diabetic patients, and she quickly realised that with the staff available they couldn't do it in the usual one-to-one way. That was when she suggested that they should teach patients in groups and organise the sessions so that the patients could help out one another. As the patients assisted one another, the specialist nurse watched them to assess who understood diet and insulin therapy.

A readiness to speculate about what is problematic, or what could be done better or differently to make the best use of the finite resources and expertise available, is often at the heart of high-quality healthcare. Even when others prefer to work within the status quo, it is incumbent upon nurses to examine what is being done – and what more could be done – to improve patient care (Bolton, 2015).

How can we reason better?

Let us take stock. So far, we have acknowledged that critical thinking is important because of the challenging healthcare environment which you will work within. We have defined critical thinking as an inquisitive but disciplined process that involves human experiences and feelings, as well as empirical information. We have suggested what the key components are within critical thinking (e.g. deciding what can be claimed) and acknowledged the aptitudes that you will need to develop (e.g. asking questions) in order to succeed. I have suggested that learning involves incremental work towards templates, that which enables us to work effectively and efficiently to address nursing care needs. What seems effortless to the experienced nurse seems difficult for us because we are still developing our thinking skills.

At this stage, it is tempting to hope for a formula, a sure-fire way to think in the right way. Would that we could use that formula to write all of our essays! Unfortunately, there is no neat formula that encapsulates critical thinking in every circumstance. You will need to reason in different ways at different times, and sometimes combine information from your different studies. In the past, nurses used to be taught bundled information (e.g. surgical nursing, medical nursing), but that did not facilitate the sort of nimble reasoning which nurses need today. We should not trap information in different silos relating to, for instance, cancer. That which we learn about coping, for example, may span cancer and many other contexts.

Nimble reasoning seems to work in two ways, sometimes in parallel:

- *Deductively*: We test working hypotheses to see whether what we predict is in fact the case (e.g. concerning how people usually cope with cancer).
- *Inductively*: We gather information in order to formulate theories of what is happening (e.g. noticing that patients tell stories about their cancer and personalise it as a means of managing stress levels).

Not all critical thinking is equal. There are certainly weaker and stronger ways of reasoning, and this usually informs how tutors mark coursework. The more sophisticated your reasoning approach, the better the mark you might attain. Rest assured, though, that expectations regarding your reasoning ability grow incrementally over the course – you are not expected to be an expert at the outset.

> ## Activity 1.7 Decision-making
>
> Look now at the descriptions of reasoning described in Table 1.2. Decide which you think are the more sophisticated forms and which are much more basic. Decide for yourself if you employ one of these approaches more than others.

Reasoning approach	Description
Independent reasoning	We construct knowledge, a template that adequately explains what is important about the work that we do. Perhaps that explains successful care: the nurse marries what the patient believes they need with what science recommends. We take a **position** on that subject.
Contextual reasoning	We rely strongly on contexts to determine what we focus upon and accept that as important and valuable. For example, we might suggest that the social circumstances of the family of a dying patient strongly influence how they cope with the news that the illness is incurable.
Transitional reasoning	Reasoning involves living with doubts, about what is true, best, defensible or important. We learn to wait and see, and accept that right now several explanations of the situation might be supportable.
Silent absorption	We absorb and appreciate a growing volume of information, contemplating the same without necessarily venturing an opinion. For example, perhaps you attend a series of lectures on physiology, venturing no opinion on what is discussed there until all of the important facts are to hand.
Absolute reasoning	We search for what is right or wrong, making clear distinctions – that which is fact and that which is not. We search for the definitive answer that properly supports care decisions.

Table 1.2 Ways of reasoning

1. Absolute reasoning

Debate continues about what represents more or less sophisticated forms of reasoning. Nursing demands different forms of reasoning at different times, but here I venture the following. The least sophisticated forms of reasoning are what Baxter Magolda (1992) calls *absolute* (Mason, 2005). At this level, the individual is unable to see the different nuances of a situation or accept that a range of possible perspectives could be taken on a subject. The thinker looks for certainty and only feels secure when matters have been decisively concluded (e.g. 'this is right', 'that is wrong', 'this is what we believe', 'that is what we don't believe'). If you are prone to thinking in this way, you might note how often you ask your tutor or practice supervisor to define what is 'correct'. While an absolute might be expected with regard to some areas of work (e.g. the right drug to use in an emergency), it is not something that is possible or even desirable in many other situations (e.g. finding the right way to deal with a hallucinating patient). We need to be more flexible in our approach. **Absolute thinking** is a common way of reasoning at the start of a university education, and it is the least sophisticated because we expect rules to govern so many things.

2. Silent absorption

I have placed silent absorption next, at least where the individual feels incapable of comprehending what the important issues are. The thinker waits, soaking up more and more information in the hope that reasoning will be assisted by the accumulation of knowledge. In practice, this does not always work out, even though it may have been your tried-and-tested way of coping. More information does not always lead to clarity, and there is a need to ask questions and discuss ideas if we are to develop confidence in our reasoning. Staying at the back of a class and hoping to avoid debates and discussions is not the best way to learn to reason, although it is understandable to begin with if the subject is entirely new to you.

3. Transitional reasoning

I suggest that transitional reasoning comes next. The thinker is ready to live with the uncertainties of knowledge but is also ready to question as opportunities present themselves. You will need to reason in this way, accepting that in some clinical contexts, and for the time being, not all can be understood about a situation. Insights emerge from what is experienced and discussed, and in the meantime it is necessary to remain alert to what experience or a carefully selected question can assist you with. You might be using transitional reasoning if you habitually try out questions with your tutor to clarify what seems defensible and important.

4. Contextual reasoning

Contextual reasoning is even more sophisticated and suggests that the thinker understands there are lots of different truths in the world – and what works in one context does not always work in another. This is not to suggest that you have no principles or standards, or that 'anything goes' within nursing. Principles and safe practice are important, but there may well be different ways of doing things within those parameters. A good example of this working well is where nurses explore with patients the nature of dignity. What represents dignified care can vary widely, and takes into account patient expectations, lifestyles and customs (Blomberg et al., 2019).

5. Independent reasoning

Independent reasoning is arguably the most sophisticated form of reasoning and one that helps you to become more innovative over time. At this level, you allow others to adopt their own position and to develop arguments in support of the same, while you build your own case about the subject in hand. You carefully search what there is to support your own position, stand ready to change it if others can persuade you, and treat all discussion in a thoughtful and enquiring way.

As you review your answer to Activity 1.7, do not be alarmed if your own thinking was near the bottom of this hierarchy. Students frequently need to work from the bottom. Moving from more familiar ways of reasoning to those that involve greater uncertainty and challenge means that you have to move out of your comfort zone. Excellent tutors are adept at helping students to do this, respecting your anxieties but always searching for better ways to help you explore nursing.

Chapter summary

I have introduced you to basic ideas about critical thinking and explained that it is a process which involves the gathering, receiving and processing of information in order to understand the world around you. It is important in nursing for a number of reasons, namely those associated with safety, creativity, problem-solving, and the management of a great deal of uncertainty that often attends patient care.

Critical thinking has a number of components that you will meet again and again. You will, for instance, have to debate what can reasonably be asserted on a given topic. To do that, you will need to develop a series of aptitudes that will help you to advance your enquiries and make more confident decisions, such as asking the right questions. These aptitudes will operate with two foci, one that deals with hard facts (empirical information) and another that deals with the human elements of care, people's feelings, hopes, values and personal identities. We must develop both cognitive and emotional intelligence.

While this can seem confusing, the purpose of your enquiries has in fact a logical and a professional end. You are learning to develop templates, ways of reasoning that work in practical and professional ways to deliver care to patients. While experienced nurses seem to do this unconsciously, they have in fact trod much the same path as you. They have learned to think, identifying patterns of information that serve them well when they deal with the ambiguity of care. There is a purpose to your learning: to respond to care requirements in an efficient, effective and patient-supportive way.

Learning to think critically, though, does not happen over night. The nursing course is designed to exercise you in different activities that help you to move from more rigid ways of thinking towards nimble and innovative ones. Learning to think critically involves some anxiety, but expert tutors and practice supervisors are well versed in helping you to find a way through.

Activities: brief outline answers

Activity 1.3 Reflection (page 16)

Here is my example. I think that we must be able to assert what counts as teaching. That might surprise you because you are learning to nurse, not to become a teacher. Yet I suggest that you will teach a great deal, especially to patients and relatives. Of course, teaching is different in clinical practice; we do not lecture patients and they are not put through exams like campus students. But we do have to help them solve problems, cope better and master medications. Knowing how teaching works, what we need to do to help patients adapt seems to me very important. It may determine whether patients stay safe and become independent again. A good understanding of teaching is of immediate benefit to practice – it has utility.

Activity 1.4 Reflection (page 17)

My memorable decision relates to helping patients recover from burns. I specialised in body image care. This patient, like many others, had facial burns and was anxious about encountering others who might stare at him. He was a Falklands War veteran who later became a public speaker, but he did not have much confidence back then. The patient and I debated how to get used to public settings again. We reviewed the merits of doing this on a 'try it and see' short-exposures basis. I suggested that he go to watch the news, sitting at the back of the ward TV room first. That was a legitimate reason to be out and about from his room but a short enough time not to become too uncomfortable. Other patients would also be focused primarily on the TV screen. I suggested that we treat it like a military exercise, with a debrief to discuss how it went at the end. We realised that to begin too quickly with more adventurous visits, perhaps to a shop or a café beyond the hospital, would seem too much. The decision, then, was a carefully consulted one, something that offered the patient options about what we might do next. I suspect that many of yours will be too. Nurses help patients to make decisions of their own.

'Nous' is a colloquial term used in many parts of the UK to mean practical common sense. A person with lots of nous knows how to get things done, with a high degree of confidence and the necessary sensitivity for the concerns of others around them. I suspect that you will meet many qualified nurses who seem to have lots of nous. Explaining to you how they reason, how they do what they do, may be difficult for some. The reasoning has become second nature and very fast. Persevere, though – if you persuade them to reflect a little bit deeper, you will have found very important information.

Further reading

Ellis, P. (2019) *Evidence-Based Practice in Nursing*, 4th edition. London: SAGE/Learning Matters.

Peter Ellis provides a tour of the different sorts of evidence, indicating the critical thinking required in order to evaluate each.

Hanscomb, S. (2016) *Critical Thinking: The Basics*. London: Routledge.

While there are a plethora of textbooks designed to help people think more critically, this one has two advantages. First, it assists the reader to challenge some fallacies in reasoning that might be presented by others. This is a valuable skill, especially as the mass media makes a range of claims about healthcare, service and quality. Second, it explores the relationship between personality and approach to critical thinking. Some individuals, for example, may be more predisposed to be open-minded about others' arguments. The textbook is not specifically directed at nurses, but it does provide an interesting extension on the introduction to critical thinking offered in this chapter.

Standing, M. (2020) *Clinical Judgement and Decision Making in Nursing*, 4th edition. London: SAGE/Learning Matters.

Mooi Standing details what underpins so much of clinical decision-making: the ways in which critical judgements are made in practice. This book provides an important illustration of applied critical thinking, drawing on ethics and evidence, as well as experience.

Useful websites

Note: Website material is subject to change or removal at short notice. The following is only indicative of valuable content.

www.wikihow.com/Improve-Reasoning-Skills

As you will see on this web page, there are a variety of things that you can do which will materially improve your critical reasoning and help you to stay alert to what nursing, and indeed life beyond, demands of you. Significantly, much of this advice holds good when stimulating the older brain, reducing the risk of dementia.

Chapter 2　Reflecting

Chapter aims

After reading this chapter, you will be able to:

- define reflection, indicating how a stated purpose can help to make reflections more critical;
- distinguish the differences between reflecting in practice and reflecting on practice, detailing why they are different from one another;
- identify six reasons why reflection is important in nursing, noting those that are most frequently used;
- discuss the best principles of reflection, identifying how you will proceed in the future;
- explain why it is important to ascertain course expectations associated with frameworks for reflection, and whether reflection should be practised at both the intimate and the skill review levels.

Introduction

Nursing is strongly associated with the skill of reflection, and for good reason. Without adequate reflection, insight and **empathy**, it would be hard to see how care could be personalised, how the needs of the individual could be adequately addressed (Price, 2019b). Without reflection, it would be difficult to see how imaginative, supportive and responsive care could be delivered over the course of a nursing career. Nurses need to understand themselves while learning to nurse, and they need to respect themselves while continuing to deliver safe care under exacting circumstances (Grigorescu et al., 2018).

While reflection is a key skill within nursing, it is not necessarily easily mastered. This is in large part because we are all accustomed to reflecting in an ad hoc way. Nursing practice reflection needs to be much better organised than that. Idle curiosity is not enough. Professional reflection needs to be characterised by several features.

First, professional reflection should have a clear purpose, one that relates to the context of your practice (Grant et al., 2017). However appealing it is to reflect in a free-ranging way, this risks confusion if the purpose of your reflection is not clear from the start. The following are some purposes that you might have for reflecting:

- To ascertain whether something represents a problem, and if so to determine why it has come about.
- To understand the process of something, such as how clinicians and families negotiate care that seems person-centred.

- To help build working templates for future practice. It is a good idea, for example, to cluster reflections around themes, such as pain management or patient history-taking. Reflections may then not only be individually more effective, but they may broaden your insight into care.

- To ascertain our strengths and weaknesses, that which sustains and motivates us in practice. Historically, reflections have been wedded to the adequacy of care, whether what you did was right. I would suggest that this is too narrow a focus, and can leave you feeling embattled and less enthusiastic about reflecting in the first place. There should be joy as well as scrutiny in nursing people.

Second, professional reflection should be disciplined (Esterhuizen, 2019). A number of reflective practice models have been developed, setting out steps to follow and questions to ask. I would suggest, however, that this is only the beginning of disciplined reflection. If you wish to reflect to a good standard, it is necessary to ask one or more colleagues to reflect with you, challenging some of the ideas that you develop. It is only by speculating with others that you will be able to fine-tune the components of critical thinking which you read about in Chapter 1.

The third feature of professional reflection relates to determining an appropriate scale for your work. The students who have influenced this book all attested to times when they attempted reflections that were too large. It is better in the first years of your studies to start with quite modestly scaled reflections, only later building up to more complex ones. You will help to manage the scale of reflection by having a clear purpose for each of them. This can also be enhanced by working with your tutor or an experienced colleague to limit the scope of the reflection. When I work with students, I remind them to limit their reflections to very discrete events, and perhaps later on to a particular stage of a patient's recovery. If the reflection combines experience and reading (something that I would recommend), then it might focus on the evidence in use. What within evidence illuminates this need or problem? What within practice highlights a gap in or strength of the evidence?

Let us begin work, then. We will look at the timing of reflection, whether we reflect in action (in the thick of things) or retrospectively upon action. We will also look at the reasoning process under way within reflection.

Activity 2.1   Reflection

Consider this statement: 'It is easier to reflect after the event rather than during it.'

- Do you support this argument?
- What premises (which we already accept as fact) underpin your position?

At the end of the chapter, I share an observation or two of my own.

Schön (1987) believes that reflecting *on* action is different from reflecting *in* action. If we reflect on the event as it unfolds, we have none of the benefits of calm introspection and time to consider at leisure the different options available to us. Conversely, if we reflect long after the event, it is likely that our memory may play tricks on us and we may remember certain features of the event better than others. Reflecting in practice involves 'thinking on our feet' (Edwards, 2017). We cannot pause the action in order to produce the sage-like response that we would love to deliver. Reflecting in action is 'raw', but it is perhaps all the more vivid for that. We can illustrate this with two short excerpts of reflection from Sue (our case study registered nurse). In the first extract, Sue is reflecting in action, and in the second she is reflecting on action. It is important to note that in-action reflections are usually unspoken – speaking aloud our thoughts could prove problematic in many clinical settings.

In the following case study, Sue has encountered a potentially aggressive relative.

Case study: Reflection in action and reflecting on action

Reflecting in action

Is this man going to hit me? He seems really angry. What does he want? I need to say something, do something that shows him I respect his concerns. I need to suggest something. I know, I'll suggest that we talk in the relatives' room but leave the door open in case I need assistance. That shows I will give him time to tell me what worries him, and I'll remain safe. Yes, that seems to have worked, he is agreeing to accompany me. But he's still talking as we go. He's like a pressure cooker, and I'm worried about how that will seem to the other relatives on the ward.

Reflecting on action

The relative had suffered a major shock. He thought he had nearly a week to prepare for his wife to come home, but she was ready to be discharged that afternoon. No wonder he was fuming. We were meeting our needs to make a bed available for some-one else but returning the patient back into his care at short notice. Colleagues could see that his wife required some more rehabilitation at home, so this was going to be a significant responsibility for him.

The above excerpts show just how different reflecting seems at these points. Notice the staccato way in which thoughts emerge when reflecting in action. There is an urgent search for meaning. Sue has to work with her perceptions of what the relative is feeling, as well as her own experiences of a confrontation. The reflections on action, however, are evaluative and confident, as well as indicating considerable empathy for the man. Sue can assert a great deal more about the origins of the problem. The important point here is that reflecting in action is necessarily less considered, less perfect than that which is possible afterwards.

In your nursing course or later as part of revalidation, you will be asked to prepare reflective practice written work. Demonstrating your powers of reflection is important. There are different levels of reflection, however – something that we discuss further in Chapter 3. What is usually sought is critical reflection, which is harder to achieve if you reflect in practice (Esterhuizen, 2019). Objective, structured clinical examinations and bedside observation examinations simulate – to differing degrees – reflection in action, but most assessment invites you to reflect on practice retrospectively. Critical reflection requires you to take an overview and understand how your own values, beliefs and goals affect the way in which you approach patients, and how that in turn interacts with how they feel and what they might wish to achieve. It is much harder to 'see the bigger picture' if you are in the midst of healthcare events.

In your course, the opportunities to reflect on practice may be legion. You will be asked to write reflective essays and develop case studies that explore the quality of care delivered to patients. Price (2017) explains how reflective practice case studies can be especially powerful, linking experience and evidence together to re-examine care. Opportunities to reflect in action and with support are much rarer. If you are fortunate, they will occur with an experienced practice supervisor who can help you to rehearse aloud your thinking within a psychologically safe environment, where a reflective account does not alarm patients (Tuomikoski et al., 2018).

It is important here to think about the sequence of events. You are likely to encounter a mass of clinical and other events (those on campus count too), which might be worthy of reflection. Manifestly, though, it is unrealistic to reflect on everything – you would quickly become exhausted. So, begin by contemplating what seems significant about your experiences. Do they relate closely to the objectives of your current module of study? Do they relate to one of your reflective purposes, perhaps something about a skill that you feel less certain about? By selecting reflections to concentrate upon, you are likely to write fewer but much better developed reflections. It is often the quality of reflection rather than the quantity of reflective records that will help to secure your progress. After all, this is a course that is designed to develop your critical thinking.

You encounter others' behaviour, which may take the form of an action (e.g. hug, shake of the fist, smile), and then you try to interpret that. But you also listen to an *account* of their experiences, feelings or attitudes (e.g. 'I'm livid that my wife has to come home from hospital without any preparation at all!'). Lying beneath that account, and either more or less coherently expressed, there may be a *narrative* – an underlying story that the individual uses to make sense of what is happening and what they are trying to accomplish (Grob et al., 2016). In this instance, the relative's narrative might relate to buying more discharge preparation time. The whole encounter, though, may be part of a bigger storyline – a *discourse* – which is something that helps to explain what is under way (Fealy et al., 2018). The obvious discourse here concerns discharge planning and lay care liaison. But it might also be about managing pressures on bed occupancy, or the need to prompt relatives to become active lay carers when this was not a part of their past role. Discourses must usually take account of your goals, values and attitudes.

When encountering an aggressive patient, you will do so with a number of attitudes already developed. It is unreasonable to assault a nurse; we are caring staff. But angry people do not behave rationally, so a primary goal is to stay safe. What we really want to achieve here is a win–win situation – one where the relative feels respected and we can find a solution to the problem of discharging the patient from hospital. Stakeholders within a discourse might disagree vehemently about what is under way and what should happen. Figure 2.1 illustrates how these elements might fit together.

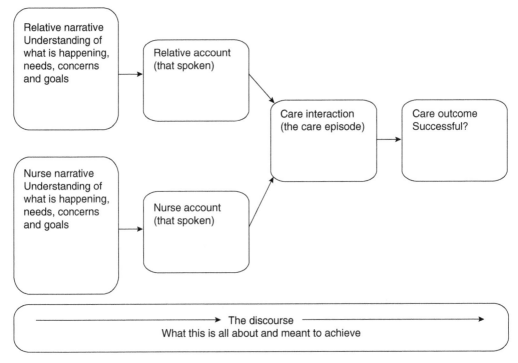

Figure 2.1   Accounts, narratives and discourses

What you learn about narratives and discourses in care is going to become very important to you. For now, the reasoning is perhaps speculative. It is difficult to be sure what you have witnessed, for now it may signal different things. You are naturally cautious. But with time, observations in clinical practice and discussion through seminars, you will develop growing confidence in interpreting what you see and hear. You will start to develop some templates that explain care in action which will enable you to approach patients in a more confident manner. You start to develop nous, the knack of saying and doing the right thing, to express care in a timely, professional and contextual manner.

Activity 2.2   Reflection

Return now to your responses to Activity 2.1, and determine whether what you have learned about accounts, narratives and discourses has helped you to understand the nurse's role in reading other people's behaviour and concerns. Can you see, for example, that both a relative and a nurse might be running different narratives to explain an encounter? Might they be promoting different discourses? Much within healthcare conflict relates to narratives and discourses, those that require gentle exploration if we are to attend adequately to one another's concerns.

At the end of the chapter, I share an additional reflection on this.

Defining reflection

Now that you have begun to explore what reflection involves, we can venture a definition:

Reflection is a process whereby experience is examined in ways that give meaning to interaction. We might examine the experience in real time or in retrospect. Because experience engages the emotions as well as reasoning, reflection needs to take account of the feelings engendered within an interaction and to allow that perceptions (how we interpret matters) may sometimes prove erroneous. While reflection is most closely associated with human interactions and especially clinical events, it is not limited to these. We may, for instance, reflect upon the written accounts of experiences, such as those shared by dying patients. Reflection may be used in the service of different purposes – those that help us to think in a more critical way and to serve the professionalism and ethos of nursing. Through an analysis of accounts, narratives and discourses, reflection helps the nurse to better understand the nature of others' needs and concerns. It may also acquaint the nurse with that which they find taxing in practice, something that must be understood if nursing is to be a lifelong career.

Why reflection is important

Figure 2.2 represents some of the reasons why reflection is so important in nursing. Your appreciation of the value of reflection is likely to grow the further you progress through your course.

Activity 2.3   Critical thinking

Study Figure 2.2 now to determine just how important reflection is to you at your current stage of studies. Is the apparent importance of reflection more closely associated with your learning or your delivery of care to others? I anticipate that you will notice a shift from the first to the second as you

(Continued)

(Continued)

progress through your modules of study. At first, reflection helps us to cope, and later it helps us to act. We begin study with a significant degree of uncertainty – what to do, how to think, where to enquire.

As this answer is based on your own observation, there is no outline answer at the end of the chapter.

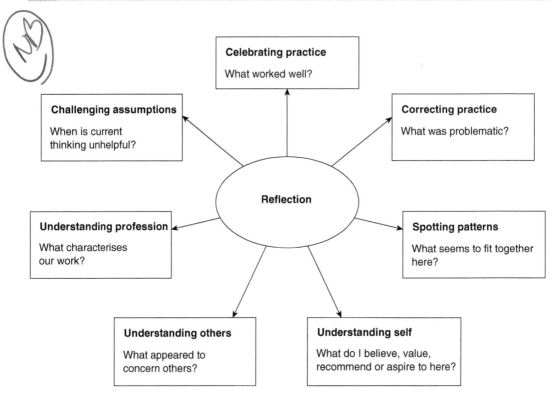

Figure 2.2 Why reflection is important in nursing

Spotting patterns

Reflection is important because it helps us to spot patterns of behaviour, combinations of evidence, and cause-and-effect events that are important in nursing (Barratt, 2019). The patterns that you might spot arise not only in clinical practice, but in classrooms and lectures as well. Themes seem to emerge and reoccur. Let me share one example with you. My clinical practice first centred on trauma, including the ways in which patients were injured, rescued, recovered and then rehabilitated. I looked after patients with burns, gunshot wounds, and bomb blast and road traffic accident injuries. Later I worked in cancer care.

One of the things that both fields of practice had in common was that they involved psychological trauma. Patients had to come to terms with changes to their appearance, as well as their body's functions and reliability. That in which they lived (the body) might not remain as comfortable or dependable as they first thought. I started to note that patients recovering from different injuries, operations and treatments seem to centre their emotional work in three areas (Price, 2016):

- managing how their body is now (the physical challenge or disability);
- revising ideals about their body and appearance or function (the body and self-esteem);
- finding ways to address the discrepancies between their body ideal and how it in fact looks or works (meeting others, feeling whole).

It seemed important to name the three areas of work (i.e. I made them into concepts). The first I called 'body reality' (the body as diseased, injured or changed). The second I called 'body ideal' (how the individual hoped that the body would seem or function). The third I called 'body presentation' (how the body is arranged, dressed and presented, that which supports self-esteem). They seemed adeaquate if not perfect shorthand descriptions. I was then able to use those concepts to focus on care work, things that I did to help the patient. So, for example, I might help a patient to rehearse new ways of thinking about themselves after a burn. What were their other atributes beyond appearance? Did people value their sense of humour, their intelligence or their compassion for others? Care was then centred on helping them to appreciate and represent themselves in a wider range of ways. This later became something that they might use to summarise their coping to others: 'My hands are burnt, but this is what I think I bring to you. I can help you to see beyond the scars.'

Do you see how spotting patterns within practice, what challenges patients, became a process of grouping information and giving each a name? Once I had done that, it was then possible to investigate what might help patients in those areas. Spotting patterns of information, behaviour, need and reaction to others assists you to theorise and eventually formulate better templates of care. While this altered body image reasoning developed over years and was large-scale, it does still illustrate the process under way. If you do not spot patterns in this way, care can become formulaic. It might seem to others that we are no longer inquisitive, and even that we have ceased to care.

Activity 2.4   Planning

Jot down now one or two themes of interest that you would like to reflect upon when you next encounter patients in clinical practice. Why are you interested in particular themes associated with one or more patients? Speculatively, what do you imagine might be discovered there? Remember that you reflect to discover – it is not a matter of simply confirming

(Continued)

(Continued)

your assumptions. Good themes to choose are those that many patients might exhibit which have practical importance for how you deliver care. These might include understanding their illness, managing treatment, asking for help or explaining their worries. The recommended reflective practice model on your course will suggest a series of questions to guide your reflection, but do not be afraid to ponder any recurring points that seem to arise from several different patients. Was a pattern forming?

As this answer is based on your own observation, there is no outline answer at the end of the chapter.

Celebrating practice

Reflection on action can be put to excellent use to celebrate practice that is success-ful and exceeds the expectations we have of it (Calhoun and Esparza, 2017). It is not enough for nurses to simply pat themselves on the back for a job well done. We need to understand how we brought about the desirable outcomes. It is easy to underestimate the value of reflection used in this role, but within a stressful healthcare environment it is vital. Reports, mass media exposés, and increasingly strident and diverse public demands made upon nurses can wear you down to the point where you debate the merits of con-tinuing. It is vital that nurses celebrate success as well as review problems and shortfalls. As you reflect on what has worked especially well in care, it is also important to consider what counts as success. Do we mean more effective care (greater impact), more efficient care (better use of resources), more sensitive care (working with the needs of patients) or more collegiate care (working better with other professions)?

While much nursing care relates to meeting measurable targets, working in concert with others to sustain healthcare protocols, you should not lose sight of the fact that of all healthcare professions, nurses are arguably among the most empathetic. Our mis-sion is to help others to deal with the experience of illness, injury or disability, as well as the problems themselves. To be empathetic is to understand how others process their experiences, how they make sense of what is happening. With this in mind, much of what is successful in nursing is best understood through reflection.

Correcting practice

Reflection is frequently used to determine what went wrong and what was problem-atic. *In extremis*, it may be used to determine who we believe was to blame for untoward events. Reflection is employed, for instance, as part of a root cause analysis (searching for the origins of a problem) in cases where there have been shortfalls in practice or a near miss (e.g. associated with a drug error) (Vincent and Amalberti, 2016). Root cause analysis gives focus to reflection and sharpens critical awareness of what went wrong. Reflecting in this way, on what was problematic or erroneous, is taxing. It is emotionally difficult to confront what we believe were our mistakes, as well as what we might have done better or differently. It becomes more problematic within a blame culture, such as in healthcare, where performances are meant to be faultless.

In some instances, what counts as a problem might seem relatively self-evident. For example, if the patient received the wrong drug and was adversely affected as a result, then that is problematic. But in some other areas of care, the decision on what represents a problem might be contested. Imagine an anxious set of parents who believe that a particular treatment might significantly improve the quality of life of their terminally sick child. For these parents, it is problematic if the clinical team do not provide that treatment. Expert evidence is called upon and relevant research is quoted. The problem is then that the definitions of both 'problem' and 'solution' become hotly contested. Nurses, as members of a clinical team, can get caught up in complaints, and this in itself raises additional problems about the stance that the nurse should take on the contested issue. Sometimes, then, reflection is used to understand why there are competing views and why the debate is stressful for all concerned.

Reflecting on what seems problematic is easier with a mentor. This individual explores with you your perceptions of events and helps you to examine the conclusions that you reach. How big a problem was this? Why did it occur? What were your options? What decisions were important here? What are the pluses as well as the minuses of the course of action that you chose? As part of her preparation work for revalidation of her practice, Sue (our case study registered nurse) described the help that she got:

> *My practice supervisor was perfect as she uses the word 'because'. She might say, 'I think that situation was a problem because the team were making different assumptions about care.' She might say, 'I think you're wrong to chastise yourself over that because the patient was very ambiguous about what they already understood about their illness.' You only benefit from reflection when it gets linked to reasoning, and a word as simple as 'because' facilitates that.*

What distinguishes an argument from mere opinion is the addition of underlying premises, those assumptions (hopefully supported by evidence) that underpin what you say (Price, 2019a). This is why the word 'because' is especially important when building an argument, presenting a discourse on how you see nursing care before you. So, in the altered body image case study above, it was important to offer evidence of how patients struggled with their disability, revised their ideals, and searched for better ways to account for their injury and new appearance.

Understanding self

In some areas of nursing (e.g. mental health, palliative care), an understanding of our motives and values is especially important because we use the self to therapeutic purpose. Our ability to share personal insights, or to imagine how others feel, may be critical (Sinclair et al., 2016). The ability to empathise, for example, becomes integral to entering the world of the patient and their anxieties, but one that must be managed with a certain detachment if professional judgements are to remain sound. A successful nurse builds an excellent rapport with patients and empathises with their concerns, but also manages to adopt a position where they can later challenge some of the patients' unhelpful beliefs.

These are important points and may be the focus for some of your study interests. If you think of nursing in craft terms, your emphasis is likely to be on skills and the way that these are selected and applied. However, if you think of nursing in more aesthetic terms, you are likely to feel more comfortable reflecting on your values and beliefs, precisely because you see these as a means to deliver the best care. In recent years, and under considerable healthcare service pressures, the values of nurses have come under increasing scrutiny. It is no longer taken for granted that nurses have a vocation and will instinctively do the right thing.

Understanding others

Much of nursing is concerned with assisting others. Person-centred care assumes that we can successfully ascertain the patient's worries, needs and aspirations as a key determinant of the negotiated nursing care (Price, 2019b). If we are to practise sensitively, then we must understand people and their backgrounds. There are some problems, though, with using reflection to understand others – chief among these is what we might call the 'common sense' fallacy. We might take it as a given that people in a particular situation (e.g. when suffering pain) will wish to proceed as we would (i.e. to have that pain alleviated). We are at risk of imagining that our preferences and wishes are shared by others and neglecting a check on their views. In reality, not all patients aspire to alleviate all of their pain; indeed, some may refuse pain relief measures altogether. A devout Buddhist, for example, might observe that pain has something to teach us, and to remove it entirely is unhelpful.

Reflection used to understand others is necessarily speculative and needs to accommodate what arises out of their situation. What is important here is the discovery of the other person's narrative, how they explain events to themselves. The fact that a person relies upon odd information, which the nurse might not view as credible, should not prompt the nurse to simply correct them. We have to understand the process of the patient's reasoning. That narrative might be reinforced by family opinion or the assessment of lay carers, and it may seem entirely unscientific. Yet until the nurse understands how the other person reasons, no individualised support can really be offered. That which might at best be considered helpful could quickly be received as a 'busybody prescription'. Reflection in these circumstances might become collaborative, the nurse assisting the patient to review what they think is happening and what needs to be done next. Where factual errors are then identified, a careful correction can be made, but in most other instances the supportive and reflective stance is one of helping the other person determine what they think now.

Understanding the profession or service

It may surprise you to discover that reflection has a part to play in understanding your chosen profession and service, and there will be opportunities within your course, as well as later within revalidation, to reflect on 'what nursing is all about'. Such opportunities provide a chance to revisit how nursing seems to change. Part of what sustains you as a practitioner concerns clear ideas about what nurses do, what expertise they bring, and what is different about the practice of the nurse. These are important considerations in a healthcare world where nurses are asked to diversify the sorts of work they engage in and where financial or other constraints might shape what the nurse can achieve (Allen, 2015).

Challenging assumptions

Reflection plays a major role in changing practice and changing profession over time. Healthcare work is not static, but it evolves, and what was once seemingly ideal later becomes suspect and anachronistic. For example, if you were to read nursing textbooks from the 1960s, you would discover that nursing care was perceived simply as supplemental to medicine. Today, nurses are much more strategic and engage in the design of healthcare (Wilson et al., 2019).

One of the best uses of reflection, then, is at a conference or when reading a report or policy associated with nursing to ascertain: (a) whether this reflects your current understanding of best practice; and (b) whether, in the light of what you have encountered there, you need to change. Reflection in this context is often best conducted as part of a group of nurses, especially where local protocols or best practice guidelines are formulated. Working in concert with others, you are more likely to formulate an informed opinion and counterbalance the first negative emotional response that can arise when you are invited to change. As a student, you may have opportunities to join team meetings and discussion groups where just such reflections are under way.

Activity 2.5   Reflection

In a seminal paper on the planning of future healthcare services, Carr et al. (2011) highlight the importance of experience, that which makes good sense of the client's needs. Research evidence, protocol and policy might have to be questioned or augmented. Imagine that you are at a conference and about to challenge a speaker who advocates change on the basis of everything but experience. Jot down three arguments that you would make to argue in favour of experience-based healthcare design, that which might be discovered through reflection.

As this answer is based on your own observation, there is no outline answer at the end of the chapter.

Arguments in favour of experience-based healthcare design might relate to client satisfaction, informed consent and person-centred care priorities. Reflection is key in each of these areas, understanding what sustains and develops services to coherent effect. Healthcare practice includes issues relating to 'could' as well as 'should'.

Making reflection work for you

Having defined reflection and made the case for its importance in nursing, I now consider how you can make reflection work for you. Table 2.1 sets out what I recommend at this stage. I then proceed to examine what is involved in association with each of the recommendations made in Table 2.1.

There are important points to make about Table 2.1. The first concerns wide-ranging reflection versus purposeful reflection. Some of the frameworks used by students to conduct and record their reflections focus solely on the episode itself. You might accumulate a large number of unrelated reflective episode records. It is then more difficult to determine what you are discovering. Start with a purpose for your reflections. By exploring the accounts of patients, relatives and practitioners, those that could influence policy, you will be better placed to examine how nurses can improve care. This is especially important as part of revalidation work for qualified nurses. The NMC requires registered nurses to record evidence of their professional update activities (e.g. attendance at a conference), others' evaluations of care, and personal reflections on practice (NMC, 2019). A much more powerful case can be made about the nurse's fitness to practise when reflections connect two or more of the different elements together. So, for example, linking reflections to patient feedback on the quality of care is a good way of demonstrating the nurse's responsiveness to expressed patient need.

Activity 2.6   Group-working

A useful reflective exercise is to focus on an area with which most of you have some experience. Most people have some experience of grief (e.g. a lost relative or friend, changed circumstances such as divorce, the loss of a pet), so this can be a good starting point from which to explore some themed reflections.

Start by individually cataloguing your perceptions of what grief is and what is needed in terms of support. Writing points down will help you to map the range of ways in which grief and support are understood.

Share your thoughts with the group. Do the points raised by others expand your understanding? If you noted some widely agreed points, does that give you confidence to start building some ideas as regards what constitutes human needs? If you collectively discover some patterns of information, so much the better.

As this answer is based on your own observation, there is no outline answer at the end of the chapter.

Recommendation	Notes
Start with a clear, reflective purpose, a question or theme that helps guide your enquiries.	In order not to end up with a mass of unrelated or difficult to relate reflections, it is a good idea to start with a theme. There is no 'right' number of reflections to complete, only clear evidence that you are deducing things from what you see and hear.
Reflect when you are fresh.	Reflection is often hard work and may provoke uncomfortable emotions. It is important to select the best times to reflect, when you feel emotionally calm, and where you have found the right space to conduct such work.
Identify confidantes with whom you are comfortable reflecting.	Choose reflective partners that you trust, not simply those who will affirm your opening assessments of events. If they say things such as 'Have you thought about …', then you have the right sort of partner.
Allocate sufficient time and attention for the enterprise.	Reflection is a meditative activity that requires as much thinking time as writing time. It is wise to allocate at least 30–60 minutes to produce one or more thoughtful reflections (i.e. those that can prove useful later).
Use a reflective practice model that fits with college requirements but do not be a slave to the questions.	You need a consistent framework to help you reflect but there will be times when the questions do not exactly fit your needs. Sometimes, for example, you will need to ask other questions to speculate how this reflection fits with others in a theme. Remember that reflection can also link what you witness to what you have read or been taught.
Create reflective records that you can use again.	To use reflective records later, you need to include enough contextual details to understand the events in question. Make sure that you remind yourself what was happening, when the events occurred, and what resources or support were available. Date the record to help you sense any changes in your perspective that occur over time.
In making and using such records, respect the rights of others.	In making reflective records, you necessarily refer to other people, so ensure that you make their names and roles anonymous. It is important to store records securely and ensure that you do not unfairly defame others. Read over your written reflections, as well as inviting others to do so, to reduce the risk that you are simply reinforcing past prejudices or assumptions.

Table 2.1   First principles of successful reflection

As well as thinking about how much time you allocate for reflecting, consider too the sequence of thinking and writing. In part, you are thinking even as you write, but this has the disadvantage that as your thoughts arrive on the page or screen, further thoughts – sometimes contradictory ones – are triggered: 'It could be this, it could be that.' 'This was important, but then again perhaps it was not.' Therefore, it seems beneficial to allow yourself thinking-only time, or perhaps 'think and jot ideas down' time, so you can play with the possibilities before you. While the final written reflection does not necessarily need to be highly polished, it should be sufficiently accessible and coherent for you to use it to revise your care later. For that reason, I advise thinking and drafting thoughts first, then penning refined reflective records later. Both spontaneous notes and final reflections can be recorded in your portfolio (offering a full audit trail of thought).

Activity 2.7   Research

Investigate which reflective framework is recommended in association with your course. Discuss with your tutor what is expected in association with each of the reflective model headings there, and whether the course permits any latitude with regard to how you set out your records. Establish whether the recommended framework allows you to state clearly the purpose of your reflection, or whether you need to add this as a preliminary introduction.

As this answer is based on your own observation, there is no outline answer at the end of the chapter.

Chapter summary

This chapter has explored reflection as a form of critical thinking, one that focuses in particular upon experience and takes into account the emotions associated with experience, as well as an account of empirical events. Episodes of care are best connected to notions of quality care through an understanding of narratives and discourses. What do people value? What do they care most about? Particular emphasis is placed on organising reflections with a clear purpose and searching for emergent patterns that might guide your future studies and even prompt you to sketch out templates of what you think is needed in such care situations.

In practice, reflection seems like two skills in one. If we reflect in action, we are thinking on our feet and reading practice situations as quickly and accurately as possible. If we reflect on action, we use the benefits of hindsight but need to beware that reflecting too long after an event can result in problems associated with memory. While it is unrealistic to analyse all experiences *in situ* (you would suffer from information overload), it is possible to accumulate reflections after events, increasing your insights into your motives and actions, as well as the consequences of what you do.

Reflection involves a process and several activities (e.g. deciding when to reflect, identifying a purpose, choosing how to frame the reflection, making a record). In support of that, I have shared a series of suggested best principles associated with this work. It is important to work with university reflective frameworks, as reflection is itself a part of the curriculum and the ways in which students are expected to learn.

Activities: brief outline answers

Activity 2.1 Reflection (page 31)

It might not surprise you that I think reflecting after the event is easier than during it, provided that there is not too great a time lag until we reflect. To reflect on events from today or yesterday is viable, but to reflect on events from a month ago is more suspect because of memory. Here are the premises that inform my position:

1. During events, we often experience information overload, and that information comes in different forms: words, sights, sounds and touch. So, to process it, to assign it meaning, is so much harder.

2. When we are in the midst of practice, we are acting a role, playing a part. So, we have to attend to what we feel, say or do, as well as what others initiate, how they in turn react to us. Reading that amount of interaction is very difficult.

3. The way in which people communicate moment by moment is often ambiguous. We can only start to make sense of an episode when we begin to identify patterns of behaviour, sequences of things said. This is because we make sense of patient wholes rather than isolated fragments of behaviour. We are much more likely to identify those when reflecting back on events. Reflecting back, we may draw on other experiences to spot what seemed important.

Activity 2.2 Reflection (page 34)

Understanding something about accounts, narratives and discourses helps us to describe what is happening in a dialogue between a nurse and a patient or their relatives. Without such nomenclature, we might simply take the other at their word, without a search for what they intended, what they hoped to convey. Imagine how a patient describes their growing symptoms over an early stage of their illness. Each symptom means little by itself – it could signal many different illnesses. But just as the symptoms start to align and relate to one another, so phrases that they share start to represent patterns about what they mean. The way in which a patient describes their symptoms perhaps tells us something about their level of anxiety and what they hope we will do. Their account of symptoms suggests something about their state of mind. We need to read that if we are to relate well to them. Over time, patients narrate their illness, creating a story of the disease that makes sense to them. We have to read that narrative if we are to seem respectful to their concerns. Of course, the other person's views may become quite polemical, a discourse about how care *should* be, how they evaluated what you did. Care is sometimes political, and that is hard to avoid in a consumer society, so we must search for any discourses in what patients say. Accounts, narratives and discourses can than help to guide what we focus upon in reflective practice.

Further reading

Esterhuizen, P. (2019) *Reflective Practice in Nursing*, 4th edition. London: SAGE/Learning Matters.

This practical guide recommends the use of reflection in a range of settings, the development of more inquisitive and speculative approaches to nursing care, and ethical ways to make reflective practice records.

Thompson, S. and Thompson, N. (2018) *The Critically Reflective Practitioner*, 2nd edition. London: Palgrave Macmillan.

Authors vary to the extent that they conceive of reflective thinking as personally therapeutic (i.e. something that helps you to cope with the stresses of practice). Sue and Neil Thompson cover both perspectives: reflection as a means to reason better (cognitive purpose) and as a means to sustain yourself (emotional or aesthetic purpose). The section on reflecting in pairs or groups is especially well summarised.

Useful websites

www.open.edu/openlearn/ocw/mod/oucontent/view.php?id=64108&section=3.2

This web page is part of the Open University's OpenLearn study skills for study, and it illustrates the difference between critical and uncritical reflection. What may interest you further is the way that reflection is conceived in different fields of practice/academic disciplines.

https://latrobe.libguides.com/reflectivepractice/models

It is extremely likely that your own university will have a web-based guide to reflective practice models or frameworks. The La Trobe University one, though, offers a selection in summary, contrasting those that are more detailed and prescriptive with those that are much less detailed and possibly less supportive for newcomers. Once you have practised reflection for a while, there is much to recommend using a simpler set of reflective questions: What? So what? Now what? But we begin in different places and you might use a more prescriptive reflective framework.

www.ed.ac.uk/reflection/reflectors-toolkit/reflecting-on-experience/gibbs-reflective-cycle

It is important to begin work with a reflective practice model recommended by your tutor and/ or university. Gibbs' model is one of the more commonly used, in part I think because it attends to both feelings and cognitive reasoning. Whether all reflections necessitate both is perhaps debatable – some might notionally concentrate on one rather than the other. Remember that models and frameworks are heuristic (i.e. designed to help you learn). They are not straitjackets that forever and everywhere define what reflection must entail.

Chapter 3 Scholarly writing

Chapter aims

After reading this chapter, you will be able to:

- summarise what we mean by scholarly writing, relating this to different levels of learning;

(Continued)

(Continued)

- discuss the key features of essay structure and how these facilitate your explanation of learning achieved to date;
- explore the ways in which past experiences of writing can shape assumptions about scholarly writing in the future;
- make a clear case for 'thinking time' when preparing to write an academic paper;
- identify areas within your own writing where there is future scope for development.

Introduction

Scholarly writing is not only a proof of learning (a product); it is also an exercise for the mind. We improve our reasoning, test our assumptions, and develop the templates we learned about in Chapter 1 through the process of writing and securing feedback, but it is not without effort. In the 1970s, Noel Burch emphasised the importance of this, describing the emotional work of learning (Adams, 2016). He referred to a ladder of conscious competence. At the bottom of the ladder, writing alerts us to things that we do not understand and makes us aware that we are as yet unskilled in dealing with that subject matter (Burch called this unconsciously unskilled). The feedback we receive on writing highlights things that we have not attended to, that which has been misconstrued. A scholar, though, builds upwards from that and becomes 'consciously unskilled'. In other words, the scholar becomes keenly aware of their shortfalls in reasoning and written expression. The writer endeavours to improve their written expression. With writing practice and good feedback, the nurse might progress to becoming consciously skilled (i.e. learning how to reason and express ideas on paper in a consistently clear way). If the nurse is more fortunate still, they might become very practised at reasoning and writing well, almost without conscious thought (Burch called this 'unconsciously skilled'). First, then, we have to confront what we do not yet know. We have to traverse through a period of time when feedback tells us that much of our reasoning seems disorderly. Competence and then apparent innate writing ability, which article writers seem to manage so easily, is achieved only after the mechanics of reasoning and writing are well understood. You can read more about Burch's theory by visiting **www.gordon training.com** and searching for the four stages of learning.

I start this chapter with three observations to reassure you. First, writing in a scholarly way is a relatively new skill for most students. Even though you may have written academic essays at school, it is less likely that these will also have been vocational work, linking theory to practice. The concepts that you dealt with there were perhaps less applied (e.g. not involving ethics or professional philosophy). Within an undergraduate pre-registration nursing degree, your thinking and writing will need to progress through different levels. Personal tutors understand this, so you should make good use of them as the assessment requirements evolve over the course of your studies. It is not 'weak' to seek guidance on meeting the requirements of your assessments. Second, writing in a scholarly way can be successfully learned provided that you take a little time to consider the process of work before you. While there are several different writing formats used within nursing courses (e.g. writing reflectively, writing about theory), all are open to analysis, and students can and do improve their writing with practice. We will return to different formats of writing in Part 3.

Stewart, Fatima, Raymet and Gina (our case study nursing students) all concede that they find writing difficult. Stewart came to nursing from a career in commerce, where his writing was less reflective than is often required here. Fatima and Raymet note that they not only wrestle with writing in the required nursing form, but also with some of the conventions of academic discussion as dictated in British universities. There were different traditions of writing where they studied before, in India and Botswana. Gina thinks that she begins with the clearest possible starting point as she is not used to any other tradition in writing. She has the most recent experience of secondary education. Their personal tutors have acknowledged the various challenges they all face, observing that students who move between one career, culture or educational system and another need help to adapt to the expectations of their new environment. Irrespective of which background students come from, then, new skills will have to be learned and past assumptions about writing reconsidered.

In this chapter, we will work with student experiences and I will lead you through different aspects of scholarly writing. This involves the connection of critical thinking and reflection to the conventions of scholarly writing. We examine the ways in which you might best represent what you have reasoned and reflected upon. We begin this work with a brief but important introduction to different levels of learning that shape course design. It is important to understand that universities classify learning in different ways, so you will need to confer with your personal tutor to understand the course expectations in the different stages of your study. Sometimes the expectations of learning in the first, second, third and fourth years of a course are difficult to distinguish from one another. Confusingly, coursework assessments may, for example, use some descriptors such as 'critically discuss' across levels of learning, so it is hard to determine what the examiners expect. However, to help you with discussions with your module leader and personal tutor, I venture my own **taxonomy** (a framework), describing levels of critical thinking and reflection that relate specifically to the applications of thinking discussed in Chapters 1 and 2. I use them here and in Part 3 to better illustrate how your thinking might become more sophisticated as a course progresses.

I next examine how best to prepare for writing. I discuss the basic structure of academic pieces of work. While this will vary depending upon the format of writing that you are asked to engage in, we believe that there are some opening tenets of good writing that can be learned here. Lastly, I discuss what we mean by **academic voice** (Price, 2003). Academic voice refers to what the student hopes to convey in a piece of writing. Some students might, for example, simply wish to flatter the tutor, agreeing with what they have taught and emulating their perspective. Usually however, you are required to develop an independent and inquisitive voice, a style of writing that critically examines what others have claimed and ventures considered arguments of your own. Understanding the style of writing required, the academic voice, will help you to write a more successful paper.

Levels of learning

While most students experience assessment work simply as a series of hurdles to be completed, universities structure work in a quite specific way. Less taxing assessments appear at the start of the course and more exacting ones towards the end. As the subject matter studied changes, this progression might not be quite so apparent to you. You may identify easy and hard subjects, which might effectively cloak what the educators are working to achieve. In principle, though, less exacting ways of thinking and reflecting are tolerated at the start of your studies, and then, when you have been taught more skills and have been practised in academic writing for longer, you are expected to demonstrate more sophisticated reasoning.

When planning courses, universities work with learning taxonomies to determine what is expected of you as you move through different levels of study. Some classic taxonomies have formed the basis of much academic thinking. In 1956, for example, Benjamin Bloom devised a taxonomy for both cognitive (reasoning) and affective (that involving emotions and reflection) learning (Bloom, 1956), work that was adjusted more recently by Anderson and Krathwohl (2001). My purpose here is not to share a history of learning taxonomies, but it is valuable to understand how they work, so Figure 3.1 shows a taxonomy used in the cognitive domain by Anderson and Krathwohl (2001).

What this diagram tells us is that it is considered much more sophisticated to understand than to remember something, and that both are bettered by being able to apply your thinking to a context. That context might be clinical practice, but it could also be a more abstract discussion of theories and policies, for example. The assessments that you complete will operate at one or another level within a taxonomy such as this, and that level can typically be spotted by the words used in the assignment question. So, for example, if you are asked to simply list and define something, your learning is being assessed at the remembering or understanding level. If you are asked to interpret something, to apply it to a practice context, your reasoning is being assessed at the application level. If you are asked to appraise or debate a subject, then you are being asked to analyse. If you are asked to design something, then you are invited to reason at the creative level. The often used 'critically discuss' assignment instruction can be confusing, because in this taxonomy 'discuss' is usually associated with comprehension and

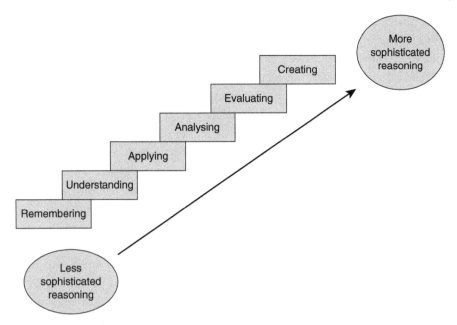

Figure 3.1 Cognitive learning taxonomy (based on the findings of Anderson and Krathwohl, 2001)

understanding, and 'critically' is usually associated with analysis or evaluation. I make the point to emphasise the importance of discussing assessment question requirements with module leaders and personal tutors.

Activity 3.1   Reflection

Look back in your course handbook to see what learning outcomes have been set for your studies, and how these change as you progress from Year 1 to Year 2, and so on, through the programme of studies. Do the learning outcomes associated with the later modules of your study seem harder? Is there a greater emphasis on creativity and the ability to evaluate?

As this answer is based on your own observation, there is no outline answer at the end of the chapter.

Reader feedback on previous editions of this book suggests that it helps students to see taxonomies of critical thinking and reflection which distinguish between different levels of achievement. Remember that these exist to facilitate your discussions with your tutors, to clarify what counts as more sophisticated reasoning and reflection. With such a caveat noted, I have ventured two taxonomies below.

I have been persuaded by Baxter Magolda's (1992) explanation of levels of reasoning, which offers a clear explanation of how reasoning can progress. In the least sophisticated forms of reasoning, individuals are inflexible and rule-governed, seeing only one explanation, one point of view. As reasoning becomes more sophisticated, it becomes first **transitional** (other possibilities are accommodated) and then contextual. The reasoning is nuanced, and it relates to a given set of circumstances. It is not that theories are not valuable; it is that they need to be understood in the context of need or use. Remember that in Chapter 1, I emphasised that it was important to discern how usable information is, whether it has practical utility. To be a successful nurse, you need to appreciate that not all information applies everywhere. You need to develop a quizzical attitude towards that which is taught: Is this true? Does it apply in every context? Ideas may seem exciting and energising, but in nursing ideas have to work with the competing demands upon the nurse. That which seems possible might not be probable when we weigh up all of the goals that we try to achieve. McBee et al. (2018) explain just how powerful and important contextual influences are in the clinician's reasoning. Much of what we must understand and do is negotiated in context. There is often no absolute right answer in healthcare, only safer conclusions and more appropriate ways forward. At the pinnacle of reasoning is independent thought. For our purposes, we can think of **independent thinking** as that which includes a vision for better practice, which shows the nurse 'thinking outside the box'. Independent thought reframes information in ways that enable the nurse to see problems or challenges afresh and to identify new opportunities.

We can link Baxter Magolda's (1992) levels of reasoning to the applications of critical thinking and reflecting, discussed in Chapters 1 and 2. I have combined these into two tables: one for critical thinking (Table 3.1) and one for reflection (Table 3.2). In studying these tables, you should anticipate that the highest-order critical thinking and reflections skills will develop in full during the later modules of your study. **Contextual thinking**, for example, cannot be anticipated until you have had the chance to apply concepts and ideas in practice. Independent thinking is often associated with project work, something that is classically used to complete a level of study or your degree as a whole. Less sophisticated reasoning is never sought but is more likely to be accommodated in the earlier modules of study. While this all might seem a little daunting, remember that we learn to reason better as part of a well-designed course. You are not expected to be an independent thinker from the outset.

Activity 3.2 Critical thinking

Study Tables 3.1 and 3.2. What do you think it will feel like to progress upwards through these levels of critical thinking and reflection? Make a note of any concerns that you might have and wish to raise with your personal tutor.

As this answer is based on your own observation, there is no outline answer at the end of the chapter.

	Absolute thinking (early learning)	Transitional thinking	Contextual thinking	Independent thinking (advanced learning)
Asking questions	Few or no questions asked, information accepted as fact.	Questions asked about whether claims are correct, whether other possibilities might exist.	Nuanced questions asked, those applying to a circumstance or need. Typically, these relate to a patient, plan or practice and its protocols.	Imaginative new questions are asked, those that reframe the topic, problem or issue in some way, liberating nurses to suggest fresh ideas.
Discriminating	There is little or no discrimination about what is right, best or proven.	Knowledge is seen as contentious in some regard and open to debate. The student writes about why something may be preferred, with reference to values, evidence and goals.	Information is interrogated with regard to its fit within a circumstance or need. Theories are applied, and concepts are examined and combined with experience to explore what works.	Judgements on best information to use are now refined, articulating a range of influencing factors that the student is taking into account. The student provides an overview of issues.
Interpreting and speculating	At best, the student selects information to include in their report of what seems defensible, true and practicable. Interpretation rarely extends to why information is important. Speculation is rarely seen at this level as the thinking is rule-governed.	Speculation is apparent as the student considers different arguments about what is important, what is happening and what is needed. The written account clearly exhibits discussion of why one option is better than another.	Interpretation involves the mixing of multiple **sources** of information, theory, research, experience and protocol. The review of information is conducted with regard to a clear purpose or goal. Speculation centres on what information can or should be used, as well as what is needed in the context explored.	Independent thinking involves adding information or ideas to a discussion that are entirely relevant but which many would not have considered. The thinker questions what is given, what is a problem or need, and what might represent a solution or opportunity. The nurse speculates about what could be possible with reference to the highest standards of professional practice.
Making arguments	The arguments of others are put forward without question.	An array of arguments are presented, showing an awareness of options. The merits of different arguments are outlined. The nurse determines which of the competing arguments is most credible.	The nurse's own arguments are advanced with context, examining what is needed, ethical, relevant, realisable and coherent. Arguments may be combined from different places in order to build a convincing case for what can or should be done now.	Strikingly new arguments are presented, showing how the nurse has conceived of information in a fresh, new way. Arguments are cogent, coherently and compellingly rehearsed so that the reader feels they have learned something important and even liberating.

Table 3.1 A taxonomy of critical thinking

	Absolute thinking (early learning)	Transitional thinking	Contextual thinking	Independent thinking (advanced learning)
Spotting patterns	Information is randomly selected and arranged with no clear connections made between factors at play. Information may be recorded simply to fill spaces in the reflective framework or model used.	Information is linked one item to another, although why or how they relate to one another remains unclear in some instances. There is a notional understanding of cause and effect, and that sometimes things simply coexist and might be caused by something else that has gone before.	Now the items are discussed not only in relation to one another, but with regard to the context in which they arose. It is understood that some patterns hold good across settings (traits), but that context can also refine how something is viewed or experienced (states).	The learner recognises complex patterns of information that are shaped not only by context and trait behaviour, but which form wholes that can be described in conceptual terms (e.g. 'This is rehabilitation because it features these things'), which can be used to recommend best fit nursing action.
Celebrating practice	The reasoning is trite. There is only one version of best practice, and why that has merit is not discussed.	Success is seen like the curate's egg – it is good in part. Focus shifts to what worked and why, but it is acknowledged that not all practice was perfect.	The nurse examines why practice succeeded, with reference to the experience of different stakeholders.	The very way in which practice is conceived, what the nurse and others are trying to do, becomes part of the discussion. Practice is understood in terms of values (those of the nurse and others), that which seems of the highest quality.
Correcting practice	Practice problems are not acknowledged; or if they are, they are ascribed to the behaviour of others alone.	Shortfalls and problems that lead to the substandard practice are recognised, including those of the nurse themselves. The reflection impresses as inquisitive and honest.	The reflection on shortfalls and problems is nuanced and relates directly to the issues that are of most concern in a given practice context. The work demonstrates how the nurse thinks about what others hoped for and sets this against what they were trying to achieve.	Correcting practice involves a critical examination of beliefs, values and attitudes, the assumptions and philosophy that might shape care delivery. Independent thinkers are brave enough to explore these more fundamental issues as part of a practice review.

	Absolute thinking (early learning)	Transitional thinking	Contextual thinking	Independent thinking (advanced learning)
Understanding self	There is little or no introspection, behaviour is often thought of as common sense.	The nurse explores questions about why they thought or acted as they did, as well as the way this affects their approach to care.	The reasonableness of the nurse's approach in a given context is now honestly evaluated. The nurse recognises that they have to understand how they negotiate care, as well as how that might or might not be suitable to the changing circumstances of healthcare.	Experience is understood as an opportunity to re-examine the nurse's own values, beliefs and attitudes. The account demonstrates the way that the nurse interrogates how these relate to practice.
Understanding others	Others are understood in stereotypical terms and usually with reference to roles (e.g. 'Patients are like this, doctors are like that').	Others are understood as individuals, and usually with a history, background or training that helps to shape how they see practice. Individuals are respected for what they experience, do or achieve.	Others are understood as participants in a situation, each with their own perceptions and opinions relating to the care under way. The account is insightful and empathetic.	Others are perceived as individuals making sense of their existence, with their own philosophy and culture or traditions. The appropriateness of care is understood in terms of helping others to meet their personal needs.
Understanding profession and service	Profession and service are understood in stereotypical terms. The nurse might 'label' what others do.	Profession and service are understood as complex, involving a lot of different contributions. Consideration shifts as to why the profession or service is as it is, as well as how and why it may be shifting.	Profession and service are understood as in transit, working with a society and patients whose needs are also changing. The fit might not be perfect, tensions are articulated, and the nurse accepts a shared responsibility in improving performance.	Healthcare service is understood as a negotiated process. Standards of practice as set by governing bodies have to be understood and interpreted soundly in the face of changing healthcare demands. There is an imaginative and committed engagement in the best standards of care.

Table 3.2 A taxonomy of reflection

Preparing to write

Having explained different levels of reasoning and reflecting, we now turn to the business of preparing to write. Every time you prepare a piece of written work, you are selecting information to share, ways of expressing yourself which demonstrate that you have met the module learning outcomes and have made progress in your reasoning and reflecting. Students are surprised by the emphasis we place upon preparation time, imagining that we compose as we write. In my experience, there is real benefit in allocating 'thinking time' before you write. This is not simply a matter of making a plan; it is about distilling your thoughts before you try to use them to represent your learning. Tutors regularly comment that they can see in academic essays where students are thinking as they write. Problems include the following:

- not answering the question set, or preparing the wrong sort of coursework;
- allocating the word count poorly within the essay (early sections getting the lion's share of words);
- material being presented in an incompletely reasoned state;
- essay conclusions falling short of requirements because students have observed many things but have never quite determined what they wish to argue;
- using others' work and representing it as your own (plagiarism is much more likely when you have allocated insufficient time to the preparation of work).

Activity 3.3   Critical thinking

I asked the case study students to each consider one of the preparations in Figure 3.2 that I think of as important in scholarly writing. Your challenge is to identify the opportunities you have to engage in such preparatory work. Where do opportunities exist to think about an academic essay in preparation?

As this answer is based on your own observation, there is no outline answer at the end of the chapter.

Coming from a different professional background, Stewart is already attuned to the need to understand the writing task set. Nursing courses include a wide variety of forms of writing and each is closely associated with reasoning in different ways. For example, if you are asked to present a case study, you will need to write reflectively but you will also need to include elements of strategy linked to care. We suggest not only that you read the requirements carefully (the assignment brief), but also that you take time to clarify any concerns and queries with the person who set the brief. Pay particular attention to the wording of assessment questions. Does the assignment brief indicate what is really required by 'critically discuss', for instance? If you fail to clarify such matters and guess the requirements, mistakes can prove costly in terms of grades achieved.

Many of you may empathise with Fatima's response about the difficulty of adopting a position within a piece of coursework. In the past, students have often been required to summarise what others have said, especially teachers. Looking back to Table 3.1 and its points on making arguments, you can see that this represents absolute thinking, and something more is typically required in an undergraduate module. Past courses may have been more pedagogical, requiring you simply to condense, to replicate others' teaching. The move from a background where you are required to demonstrate what has been taught to you to one where you must reason more for yourself is difficult for students (Magnusson and Zackariasson, 2018). In my experience, this is heightened where students are required to 'take a stance on an issue' of their own. For example, in rehabilitation, where work is shared with patients and lay carers, you might be asked to state what represents a reasonable level of input by patients and their relatives. What do you expect patients and their relatives to learn and do, and what do you think nurses should contribute? In these and similar matters, you do need to make a case, and it is important for you to be completely clear about this before you start.

In Figure 3.2, Raymet's points are important: students often wonder when an argument becomes a fact. Moreover, if you are to grapple with a series of arguments, how should they best be arranged?

In nursing courses, it is often necessary to present a series of arguments, each of which supports the case or position that we adopt. You will often find within UK universities that the case or position is stated early within the academic paper, with the main text then used to rehearse arguments and counterarguments, which help the student to sum up insights within their conclusion. There are other approaches within reflective writing, which I explore in Part 3. Such essays are typical of what tests transitional or contextual thinking (see Table 3.1). For example, your case or position may be that nurses should educate patients to take on self-care activities. Arguments in support of this include: (a) patients gain independence through their own learning; (b) it is not economically viable to go on delivering all of the care, so patients and relatives need to develop their own skills; and (c) patients develop greater self-esteem through the process of learning to care for themselves. This may or may not be your experience of previous learning, where perhaps you revealed your position incrementally at the end of your paper. However, the case-first sequence is the reasoning norm for more philosophical essays within nursing, so if you have difficulties making that transition, it is worth discussing the adjustments you are trying to make with your personal tutor.

Gina is correct that tutors envisage students using a variety of resources as part of their academic writing, and that it takes time to select what will be included in a piece of coursework. Observations from practice, arguments articulated by others in interview, and hospital care philosophies are just a few of the things that could support what you write about. It takes time to evaluate each of these and judge how each resource will be linked to the arguments made (e.g. 'This supports my argument, that reminds us that there are alternative perspectives').

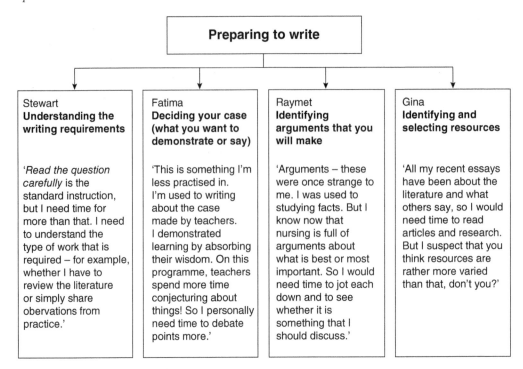

Figure 3.2   Preparing to write

Avoiding plagiarism

Plagiarism is the use of other people's written work, figures, tables or diagrams, and the representation of these as your own work within an academic paper (Pears and Shields, 2019; Price, 2014). Plagiarism carries severe penalties at university. At the least, you may receive a written warning; at worst, you may have an academic paper failed or you could be dismissed from the course altogether. It is therefore vital to prepare for writing in ways that limit the risk of committing plagiarism. Each of the following represents good preparation:

- Find and read very carefully the university rules and regulations regarding the correct representation of the work of others within your academic essays. This can usually be found within the course handbook or the study skills section of the course web page. Make a point of asking your tutors about anything that you do not understand.
- Use a notebook to record all the sources of information that you have used, including websites. Do this immediately when you find helpful material. Make a note of the website address (its URL) so that you can find it again. One of the temptations is to use notes made from websites, and then – because you cannot find the reference details later – to represent the words used as your own.
- Do not assume that because there is no author's name evident on a web page, it does not need to be referenced. The default position should be that where author

details seem to be missing, you should treat the organisation that runs the web page as the author of the work.

- Get into the habit of using quotation marks regularly at the start and end of a passage of copied words. If you **paraphrase** work (i.e. rephrase the points in your own words), make sure that you do a thorough job. Changing just the odd word within the sentence does not constitute paraphrasing, and you may be told that you have plagiarised the work. Imagine that the original text that you read said this: 'Rehabilitation is both an educational and a support process, one in which the patient is required to actively engage and one which requires the nurse to strategise, evaluating how well the patient is doing.' You might paraphrase this as: 'Nurses work strategically with patients, teaching and supporting them, adjusting rehabilitation work as they go.' The paraphrase captures the essence of what has been written without using the same words. You still then need to acknowledge the source, indicating the author's name and year of publication within brackets in the text.

- Reserve enough thinking time before you write. However daunting it seems, you do have to decide what you think about others' reported work. Examiners respect that your points will not always seem profound, but they do need to understand what sense you make of that which has been reviewed.

- Do not share essay drafts or past assignment answers with other students. There is a risk that others may copy your work and you could be charged with aiding and abetting them (academic collusion). Universities use software that can show the similarities between student work received, including that which was submitted in the past.

- Do not be tempted to purchase essay work from the internet. Not only is this considered a calculated effort to cheat (one mandating a severe penalty), but you may also be using something that is in any case not fit for purpose. Tutors are keenly aware of what you have written in the past and what this essay requires, so subterfuge essays are often spotted.

- Check to see whether your university offers you access to a script-checking service such as Turnitin (**www.turnitin.com**). Turnitin compares passages of your own work against that which exists within other published and website work, showing you where your words match those elsewhere. There is no problem with found matches where you have attributed the source of the material and used quotation marks appropriately; but where sentences or longer passages of your work match those from elsewhere and no attribution is recorded, vital corrections need to be made.

The basics of structure

Pieces of academic work have a beginning, a middle and an end, and must seem complete and coherent. It is this quality of completeness and coherence, together with authority, clarity and precision, that we search for when planning a paper. Completeness and coherence are supported by the way in which we structure the written work, authority is determined by how we present and support arguments, and clarity and precision are affected by how we help others to navigate the paper, as well as through the way in which we decide what to include and what to leave out. If we force too much information into an essay, clarity suffers.

Activity 3.4 Research

To help you explore structure more fully, select an article published within a nursing journal and read through it, noting how it is structured. Pay particular attention to the way that sections are set out and what sorts of things are discussed in each section. While published works are more polished than those submitted for coursework assessment, they nevertheless include relevant structural features that we can discuss.

When you have finished reading your chosen article, answer my questions at the end of each of the following sections.

As this answer is based on your chosen article, there is no outline answer at the end of the chapter.

Introducing the work

All pieces of academic work need an introduction, which has four roles:

- to identify the subject matter of the written piece;
- to secure the reader's attention and interest;
- to establish the writer's position or perspective;
- to set any contexts within which the paper needs to be understood.

It is possible to establish the subject matter by stating the essay question set or to simply say at the outset, for example, 'This essay is written about the rehabilitation work of the nurse.' However, there are slightly more adventurous ways of introducing a subject. An academic essay is not journalism, but like journalists we are required to interest our readers in the essay's subject matter, even if they are examiners and are being paid to read our work. We need a 'hook' to encourage them to read on. Two common ways of doing this are:

- Start with a bold point that highlights the importance of the subject matter (e.g. 'There is at least anecdotal evidence that nurses and patients are not always working to the same ends during rehabilitation').
- Introduce a dilemma that needs to be addressed (e.g. 'There is a problem with patient rehabilitation, and this is linked to what we consider ideal and what seems possible given resource constraints').

You will need to decide whether your introduction will be presented in the first person singular (referring to 'I') or in the third person, referring to 'the nurse' or 'nurses'. First person singular is the norm where any form of reflective writing is required. Where in the third person you refer to 'the author', it is important to be aware of literature review traps – are you referring to the author of other papers reviewed or to you, the author of this essay?

If your work concerns practice or an area of professional discourse (e.g. applied science, pharmacology), your introduction needs to make this clear. You might, for instance, refer to a client group to whom your work concerns (e.g. post-operative patients) or a particular area of practice (e.g. the use of analgesia).

Activity 3.5 Reflection

Examine your chosen article to establish whether the introduction achieves all of the aims of an introduction, as listed above. If any of the key features are missing, what are the implications for the rest of the piece? Look back to Table 3.1 to examine what the introduction offers as regards levels of critical thinking. Can you see how setting out a case early on, focusing the essay, might help you to demonstrate clear arguments and show how you are interpreting a subject?

As this answer is based on your own observation, there is no outline answer at the end of the chapter.

Signposting the work

Towards the end of the introduction to your work, you need to help the reader understand how the rest of the work is set out (e.g. 'This essay is set out in the following sections ...'). Signposting is not only a description of the rest of the work, though; it frequently includes an indication of the stance that you take and the purpose of your paper. You may indicate, for instance, that this paper on rehabilitation nursing considers the role of the nurse in section 1 and the role of patients and lay carers in section 2, and then debates the liaison work between the two groups in section 3 (e.g. 'The paper makes the case that rehabilitation is a negotiated activity and one that requires careful liaison between stakeholders').

Activity 3.6 Critical thinking

Did you spot signposting in the work that you chose to read? It frequently consists of just one very important paragraph at the end of the introduction. Does the signposting within your reviewed work help you to read forward with a clear purpose, knowing what the author is trying to do?

As this answer is based on your own observation, there is no outline answer at the end of the chapter.

Developing the main body of the work

Classically, academic essays include a main text with few subsections, and they rarely include figures or tables. Within nursing, however, the conventions are rapidly changing, and it is usual to arrange the work using subheadings to help the reader navigate your work, as well as including both figures and tables where these help you to make a point quickly and clearly. Check your course handbook to establish the local norms. My own preference is to encourage writing that helps the reader to follow your arguments and includes features that are similar to those used when writing for publication (e.g. section headings, figures and/or tables).

What remains important in academic papers is that you write in disciplined paragraphs, with short sentences that enable you to make clear points. Where you do use figures, tables or appendices, they must all be clearly referred to in the text and within brackets (e.g. 'see Figure 1', 'Table 3 refers to ...', 'see Appendix 1').

What do I mean by a disciplined paragraph? In practical terms:

- It attends to a single subject (e.g. ascertaining the patient's readiness to rehabilitate).
- It includes clear points and your own or others' arguments (e.g. 'While economic pressures exist to speed up rehabilitation, the readiness of a patient to learn skills still affects the pace of their progress').
- It provides support for what has been stated. This is often where references to the literature come in, but – as we have noted – other evidence gleaned from practice could be referred to (e.g. 'An example patient helps to make the case. Mr X reported that he felt paralysed by fear regarding taking exercise after his heart attack. He worried that staff had not completely understood the risks.').

Sentences that extend beyond a couple of lines of text are much more likely to seem ambiguous to the reader. Being scholarly does not necessarily mean writing longer sentences or cramming more information into a paragraph.

The last key consideration regarding the main text is that you build a series of arguments. To demonstrate that you are thinking critically, it is important not to accept points at face value. For this reason, a paragraph that makes one argument could, in some instances, be followed by another paragraph that makes a second argument. But it is important by the end of your work to demonstrate that you have reached your own conclusions, even if this is only to suggest that the debate continues. Remember that in transitional and contextual reasoning, you will have to demonstrate possible arguments and review their merits. You will need to determine the best fit arguments to a context of interest, whether that be clinical practice or perhaps a review of nursing theories and their ease of use. So, turning once more to our example, we might spend one paragraph arguing the above point about the importance of patients' readiness to commence rehabilitation and then add a second paragraph which reminds the reader that prolonged inactivity increases the risk of post-myocardial infarction complications. On balance, then, the recommended way forward is physical rehabilitation and consistent psychological support while patients test their limits.

Activity 3.7   Critical thinking

Examine your chosen article to identify some examples of what you think are especially successful paragraphs and to list the arguments you can see being developed within the main text of the paper. How does this structure compare with some of your own past essays? Can you see how the work starts to have a bigger impact on you because of its structure?

As this answer is based on your own observation, there is no outline answer at the end of the chapter.

Reaching a conclusion

Academic coursework (unless otherwise instructed) requires a conclusion. Within the conclusion, there should be no substantial new material. Its purpose is to sum up what has been written so far. However, the essay has to show what sense has been made about the arguments presented. Beyond all those points about helping the patient rehabilitate, what does this amount to? The author needs to deduce what the arguments support. Perhaps it is first to support patients because they are doing a lot of the rehabilitation work. Perhaps it is to coordinate rehabilitation work. Perhaps it is that if physiotherapy is given before patient education has been delivered, patient anxiety might be increased.

Activity 3.8   Critical thinking

Scrutinise your chosen paper to see whether the conclusion achieves the above. Do not be surprised if you identify some shortfalls here – even published papers sometimes include weak conclusions. Did the conclusion make reference to a case that was stated at the start of the essay or article?

As this answer is based on your own observation, there is no outline answer at the end of the chapter.

Adopting the right voice

We come at last to the business of 'voice'. You might be surprised that I use a term more associated with singing to describe scholarly writing. By voice, I mean conveying your thoughts in such a way that your thinking is demonstrated as something that seems orderly, measured, critical or reflective, as the need dictates. Academic voice helps you to portray that you are thinking at a higher level of critical thinking. Singers use a voice to convey emotions or drama. Students need, through their texts, to use a voice to illustrate or represent their learning. We have already conveyed two ways in which your work will seem more scholarly: first, developing a coherent structure for your work; and second, building a series of arguments that demonstrate your reasoning. There remain, though, some important niceties in the ways in which you write (i.e. use your voice) that will enhance your reputation as a scholar.

Activity 3.9   Critical thinking

Look at some sample sentences that the four case study student nurses used in their earliest essays. They are at pains to remind us that their work has improved since! There are some classic faults within these short extracts that demonstrate less than scholarly work, and I invite you to identify them.

Gina: That patients wait, lying on trolleys within a corridor or a corner of casualty, is utterly appalling.

Stewart: Time is money, so the doctor's stay at the bedside is always short and patients ask others what has then been decided as regards their treatment.

Raymet: The assessment I made of the patient was holistic. I examined their rash and listened carefully to their anxieties.

Fatima: A tutor has explained that patients sometimes only want to please the nurse, rather than state their real concerns. This seems right to me.

My answers to this activity are included in the text below.

Did you spot the fact that in Activity 3.9, Gina was using hyperbole (i.e. accentuating a point made in a heavy-handed or excessive way)? While we might share dismay at the length of time patients wait to secure a bed, and would not commend long waiting times and uncomfortable conditions, the conventions of academic writing are that we express opinion in rather more measured terms. In this example, a more measured critique of this situation might be to observe that the lengthy waits were undignified and that they raised questions about service standards. The phrase 'utterly appalling' appeals to the emotions of the reader rather than their intellect, and we do not convey analysis so clearly. A scholarly voice is measured and resists hyperbole. For example, when evaluating practice, 'the care had specific benefits', not 'the care was simply fantastic'.

Stewart's fault in this example concerned what we call a colloquialism (i.e. a form of shorthand writing that we assume the reader understands). 'Time is money' is a well-known aphorism that describes how people prioritise their time using economic considerations. But used in this context, it hardly does justice to the doctor. 'Time is money' does not do justice to the matter and conveys the (unintended) message that some matters are obvious and can quickly be dismissed in an academic essay. Colloquial language often conveys the sort of absolute thinking seen in Tables 3.1 and 3.2.

The fault in Raymet's writing is rather more subtle but is nonetheless a good example of where the academic voice has not yet been developed. If work is to be precise, it is necessary to use terms and concepts with care. In this instance, Raymet is referring to holism and claiming that the assessment of a patient was holistic. However, 'holistic' refers to four major aspects of a person's life and experience: the physical, psychological, social and spiritual. It suggests that the care delivered engages deeply and comprehensively with the patient's experience (George et al., 2017). What Raymet reports here is not a holistic assessment of the patient, but one that concentrates upon the patient's rash (physical) and anxieties (psychological). Checking a dictionary can help to resolve this issue.

There are two possible problems with the academic voice in Fatima's extract. First, there are usually conventions associated with the referencing of sources, and here Fatima is not following them. If she has been encouraged to include personal discourses with a tutor within academic work, it is necessary to state in brackets the nature of that (e.g. 'personal email communication with tutor X'). Second, students sometimes present work that is designed to please the marker of the finished work. They may refer with approval to what the examiner has taught, said or written elsewhere. In scholarly writing, though, examiners wish to learn what the student has reasoned rather than what the tutor has taught. It is necessary to demonstrate your own judgement and evaluation of issues rather than to simply approve those that you think might please someone else.

Thus, a scholarly voice is one that:

- acknowledges the source of points and perspectives of others (in the literature or elsewhere);
- demonstrates your own reasoning and reflection;
- uses terms precisely and consistently;
- expresses points in a measured rather than emotive way;
- avoids forms of shorthand reasoning such as colloquialisms.

Chapter summary

I return to the matter of scholarly writing again in Part 3. It is important here, however, to acknowledge the above precepts of good writing, some of which can seem implicit rather than explained within the course that you study. Pausing to consider

(Continued)

(Continued)

what is required of you by your tutor and the university, as well as where that fits and does not fit with what you have learned before, can help you to understand what seems more challenging about study. Most of what is required is determined by the need to convey your learning in as clear and accessible a manner as possible: by adhering to simple practices, by writing a paper that has a clear beginning, middle and end, and by using devices to guide the reader through the work. It is about considering how much information you can or should include within a sentence or paragraph, as well as whether your work within that paragraph has strayed away from its subject. It is certainly about good spelling and grammar, as well as checking work before it is submitted.

Of all the fundamental errors in scholarly writing that I see within nurse education programmes, there are three which recur frequently. Some students fail to appreciate what sort of writing they are asked to provide. Like Stewart, they need to clarify the requirements set, usually by taking questions to the tutor. Other students begin to write long before they have concluded what they think. Tables 3.1 and 3.2 emphasise just how important and complex thinking can be. Students are then hard-pressed to identify what case they wish to present. 'Thinking time' is more important than 'writing time' and it is worth investing in, especially if you jot down notes about your developing ideas. A third group of students rush forward with their writing, failing to attend to the academic voice required within assignments and using imprecise colloquial terms. The net effect is that their work seems ill-considered and hurriedly prepared.

Many of the papers that students have criticised as 'too descriptive' are associated with such faults. Arguments are lacking and the ideas discussed have been handled in a shorthand way.

Examining examples of scholarly writing in different places will help you to identify what conveys learning clearly and well. By studying the resources that you find within the university library, you will be much better placed to represent your reasoning and reflection when it comes to work that carries course marks.

Further reading

By definition, I see a need for a book on reasoning, reflecting and writing in nursing (this one). There are, however, some other texts that I admire on the more general principles of essay-writing. You are recommended to look at these if you wish to augment that which is offered in this book.

Greetham, B. (2018) *How to Write Better Essays*, 4th edition. London: Palgrave Macmillan.

This is an accessible and logical guide to the business of finding information and making coherent notes, as well as turning these into coherent and adequately source-cited essays.

Pears, R. and Shields, G. (2019) *Cite Them Right: The Essential Referencing Guide,* 11th edition. London: Red Globe Press.

Time spent investigating plagiarism at the Open University taught me just how easy it is for students to misconceive referencing requirements, so an additional resource on this topic (beyond your university guide) is not a bad idea.

Price, B. (2017) How to write a reflective practice case study. *Primary Healthcare,* 27(9): 35–42.

There is a paucity of guidance on how to write well by combining both experience and evidence together. Yet this is just the sort of practice-relevant, evidence-rich work that is arguably required in nursing. Case studies are a good way of combining the two. This article explains how to structure a piece of writing clearly, establishing why the topic is important for your readership. Price argues that case studies also have merit when preparing evidence of learning for revalidation purposes.

Useful websites

Each university produces its own guide to good academic writing processes and sets out requirements for the way in which assignments should be presented. Conventions may differ by university. I therefore direct you to the study skills section of your university website rather than prompting you to a wider trawl of the internet.

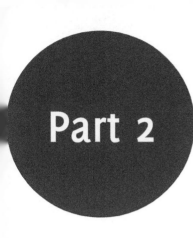

Part 2　Critical thinking and reflecting in nursing contexts

Chapter 4 Making sense of lectures

Chapter aims

After reading this chapter, you will be able to:

- detail ways to engage in a lecture so as to enhance the quality of your learning;
- summarise ways in which to prepare for a lecture;
- discuss the different ways of thinking in a lecture that might enrich your experience;
- explain why questions are so important to learning in a lecture;
- summarise important things to do after a lecture has ended.

Introduction

In skilful hands, a healthcare lecture is an inspiring experience. Higher education has moved on from the use of lectures to simply deliver information; increasingly, they are used to facilitate reasoning (Hong and Yu, 2017). Here are two ways in which our case study nursing students have experienced lectures in fresh and relevant forms:

1. Students were asked to read three seminal papers on risk-taking behaviour and how it might affect patient attitudes to healthcare guidance. The purpose of asking students to read first was to deliver the bulk of information-sharing in an efficient

way. The lecture then concentrated on how risk attitudes could be identified and how different approaches could be used to help patients make better choices in support of their well-being.

2. The lecturer presented a case study from practice, one that posed a series of ethical dilemmas for clinicians. The case study was vividly portrayed, with enough detail to assure the students of its authenticity. Then the students were led through a series of decisions about what to prioritise when approaching care. The students voted (using colour cards) which choices they would make, and the lecturer then revealed the outcome that might follow.

I hope that you agree with me that the above sessions hardly seem dull. Each prompted a great deal of critical thinking on the part of the student audience.

What is important, however, is that you pause to consider your approach to the forthcoming lecture. Raymet (one of our case study students) reflects here on some student attitudes that she thought less beneficial:

> *Some students come to lectures to simply record what the lecturer has said. They are eager to get the handout first and that's about it. I doubt that they have thought very much for themselves, at least while the lecture was in progress. Some other students try to score points against the lecturer. They delight in posing difficult questions, as though they were journalists asking questions of politicians.*

I wonder whether you agree with me that neither of the student types which Raymet describes is using lectures to best effect? The first student type is too passive. If all the student is to do is record what the lecturer argues, then it is debatable whether useful connections are then made to practice, to their own experience of the subject. The second student type is playing an egoistic game of 'beat the lecturer'. Asking questions is a good idea, but their purpose should not be to secure answers that the student barely listens to.

While some lectures are designed to present facts, policies, rules and standards, the majority are designed to offer a summary of information and possible ways to think about it. It is comparatively rare that a lecturer takes an entirely didactic approach to a subject – healthcare is too complex to encourage that (Kitson et al., 2018). A better attitude to approaching a lecture is then to try to understand how the lecturer portrays a subject, to appreciate what is focused upon and why. It is then a good idea to reflect on whether this surprises us. In short, it is wise to approach the lecture with an inquisitive frame of mind (Takase et al., 2019).

In this chapter, I assist you in planning for forthcoming lectures, as well as arriving at each with an inquisitive state of mind. I describe the features of typical lectures, as well as identifying how best to arrive at a balance between listening, thinking, writing and communicating. I finish the chapter with some work that you should undertake after the lecture has ended.

Activity 4.1   Reflection

Begin now by recalling a particularly successful lecture that you enjoyed. Identify what seemed to make the lecture such a success. Was success determined largely by the skills of the tutor, the contributions of the students, or a mixture of the two? What do you deduce from your part in that?

As this answer is based on your own observation, there is no outline answer at the end of the chapter.

Preparing for the lecture

Above, I have recommended that you approach the lecture inquisitively. You might well wonder how to do that. I have found it helpful to recommend coming to the lecture with a series of opening questions noted on an opening page in your notebook. It is then easy to refer to the questions just before the lecture begins. The questions are not necessarily the only ones that will seem relevant as the lecture progresses, but they will help to get you started by focusing your attention and prompting reasoning. The questions now follow.

Context

What is the context of this lecture and why is it important? Imagine a lecture delivered on cross-infection control and hygiene. At the time of writing, a global coronavirus pandemic is under way (Covid-19), one of a coronavirus series that has blighted humankind over the decades. Previous epidemics included severe acute respiratory syndrome (SARS) and Middle East respiratory syndrome (MERS). What is significant is that each has varied with regard to its ease of transmission and ability to incapacitate or kill (Cui et al., 2019). This affects the perception of risk and adherence – or otherwise – to preventative measures.

Connections

What seems to connect with the anticipated subject matter of this coming lecture? Lectures often operate in family groups, as it were. A lecture on ethical theory relates closely to professionalism. They are in a subject matter family of professional etiquette. Ethics highlights professional responsibilities but also raises some challenges as regards practising well. Ethical responsibilities (patients' rights) may compete with one another (Sokol, 2018). Identifying some connections in subject matter might remind you of some personal learning needs that have discomfited or concerned you. Connections are very important in healthcare. In research, for example, we often search for what correlates to a phenomenon (e.g. the aggressive patient) in order to better analyse how problems develop. A correlation is something that happens – positively or negatively – alongside other things, and it might or might not be influential in shaping outcomes (McLeod, 2020).

Causes and consequences

How do you think the lecturer will treat causes and consequences in this lecture? In nursing, both are vitally important. Much of our time is spent trying to understand causes and to anticipate – and in some instances avert – consequences. Most lectures have something to say about causes and consequences, even when they are not about diseases and healthcare problems. For instance, if you attend a lecture on the needs of the destitute, then it is worth cueing yourself in to the lecture by wondering in advance what leads people to such precarious circumstances. How do different circumstances lead to someone sleeping on the street? Consequences of destitution (in this example) are equally interesting to speculate about. For example, how do you ensure continuity of care if the patient has no fixed abode?

Caring

Nursing is fundamentally about caring in a professional, effective and efficient way for others (Ko et al., 2019). So, what might the anticipated subject matter of this lecture mean for caring? Let us imagine that the lecture is on psychoses and the ways in which these alter the perceptions of patients. What might it be like to care for a psychotically ill patient who suffers from delusions or hallucinations? How could that affect how they understand our words and behaviour? What might it mean for care planning with them? Anticipating the care implications of a lecture is a good way of piquing interest in subject matter; sometimes it leads us to questions about the feasibility of recommended care approaches.

Activity 4.2   Reflection

Imagine for a moment that you attend a small group teaching session where you anticipate a visiting speaker. The session is on psychological insecurity and how it affects patient behaviour. The teaching room chairs have been arranged in a large circle. There is no lecture podium, no screen on which to project slides. The learners assemble from several different courses, so you do not know them all. No lecturer appears. None is introduced. After some anxious conversation about whether the lecturer will turn up, the visiting speaker reveals herself among you. She was seated in the circle all along. She invites you to begin by speculating how that felt. What might it teach you about insecurity?

What do you think this visiting speaker was doing? How useful is it to experience the subject matter of a session (wherever safe)? Do you think that anticipatory questions might have helped you to respond more effectively in a session such as this?

I have offered a reflection or two of my own at the end of the chapter.

Engaging with the lecture

In the previous section, I suggested some preparatory questions that we can use to set our radar for what the lecture might have to offer. It is now time to consider how we can usefully build upon that to engage effectively with the lecturer. Engagement here refers to three key activities. First, show the lecturer that you are attending to what they are sharing (Ko et al., 2019). If you spend your entire time with your head down taking notes, then it is much less likely that the lecturer will feel you are considering their points. Lecturers depend on the visual cues that you share through your facial expressions. Just how far – and how fast – they progress with their points depends on you honouring them with an attentive gaze. Do not worry if you frown – all information of this kind signals something useful to the lecturer.

The second activity relates to the questions that you and your fellow student nurses ask the lecturer. While a lecturer may have an agenda as regards what they wish to convey within the time frame, no thoughtful teacher rejects sincere questions. Your learning is at least as important as their exposition, but you will need to agree with your lecturer the best times to ask questions. Sometimes these are taken at the end of the session. The lecturer wants you to appreciate a whole idea before debating what that means. Often, however, question opportunities are punctuated at key points within the session. This is particularly important where the lecturer builds an idea for you to study. You are asked to consider a series of arguments that add up to something bigger. You are theorising with the lecturer. Forming those theories, and perhaps even reaching a template for practice, however, is only possible if you check your understanding en route.

The third activity is responding to the lecturer's own challenges. Classically, these are posed in the form of questions that the lecturer invites the audience to offer answers to. But some lecturers are yet more skilful, and they set up provocative statements, those that you are invited to debate (Wolff et al., 2015). Of course, if you are sitting with your head down making notes, some of those may pass you by. The lecturer may want to dissuade you from simply accepting the arguments of others without question. So, listen carefully for any seemingly provocative arguments that the lecturer might offer up to you.

Discussion with your lecturer, as well as possibly with other students, deepens your understanding of key issues. It may certainly help you to remember points that could be raised later in a piece of coursework. It is in teaching sessions such as lectures that you learn to enquire, and in some measure – depending on the format of the lecture – to question and debate. Remember that in Table 3.1 (page 53), higher levels of critical thinking are associated with asking how arguments fit with contexts. So, asking questions about whether the espoused ideas work in practice is extremely important. It is necessary to ask yourself, and perhaps the lecturers too, what conditions would have to prevail before an argument made were true. Imagine that your lecturer was sharing with you some of the rights that they believe underpin nursing care. The patient has a right to confidentiality, but you remember that care is often delivered in communal environments where medical rounds are completed. So, a question about possible challenges and compromises to the right of confidentiality is entirely reasonable: 'I noted your points about confidentiality, but what about medical rounds and the discussion of problems at the bedside? Is this a problem?'

We need to ruminate on what has been said by the lecturer. If you are ready to explore how the claims made by the lecturer affect your current values, beliefs and attitudes, you are beginning to engage with the highest possible level of reflective thinking, described in Table 3.2 (page 55). Imagine that the lecturer, in answer to the last student question, contends that of necessity, nurses sometimes have to compromise on patient confidentiality commitments, as illustrated in ward rounds. How does that make you feel? Perhaps it seems a 'cop out'? Perhaps sensitive information could be discussed away from the bedside? Perhaps you think that significant and intimate information can and should be discussed elsewhere, moving mobile patients to a consultation room?

Activity 4.3   Reflection

Look now at your notebook to see how you arrange notes in lecture sessions. What gets recorded there and then, and what (if anything) is written up later? How extensive are your lecture session notes? Thinking back to Chapter 1, as well as what you have already read about theorising and the discovery of templates, what advantages can you see in building notes after the lecture has finished? We will turn to note-taking shortly, but for now I encourage you to examine what you do already.

As this answer is based on your own observation, there is no outline answer at the end of the chapter.

Typically, a lecture will include:

- *scene-setting and context-relating* – the tutor asks students to focus on a particular subject matter, often linked to lecture goals or objectives;

- *exposition* – the tutor summarises points discovered through research, presented as theory or indicated by experience;
- *illustration* – the tutor sometimes draws on their own personal experience of nursing or that shared by other practitioners;
- *speculation* – the tutor debates issues or different expositions (e.g. two or more theories of counselling may have been shared, and the tutor considers the relative merits of each);
- *interrogation and consultation* – the tutor invites responses from students, either to check their understanding or to engage them further in the subject matter;
- *summation* – the tutor sums up what the lecture has conveyed;
- *next direction* – the tutor suggests what further work, reading or reflection is now useful.

We can link the different elements of a lecture to the opening questions that you brought to the lecture (see Table 4.1).

Features of the lecture	Links to opening questions
1. Scene-setting and context-relating	Was the lecturer's starting context as you anticipated? If it was, you might feel gratified, but do not worry if it causes you to think again.
2. Exposition	The exposition might suggest new connections to other subject matter that you had not considered. It might challenge your opening ideas about how events unfold (cause and effect). The exposition might clarify what is involved in caring (e.g. the emotional work of the nurse when a patient is extremely ill).
3. Illustration	Illustrations shared in lectures tend to qualify or expand upon theory, so it is worth revisiting your ideas about contexts and how they shape practice. For instance, do all diabetic patients learn self-care in the same way?
4. Speculation	Accomplished lecturers think aloud and permit you to speculate with them. In my experience, this often centres upon the practicalities of caring, that which seems most acceptable to patients and families and which is realistic regarding resources available.
5. Interrogation and consultation	The lecture may raise issues of controversy, areas where different philosophies or schools of thought compete (e.g. in research). Care is experienced in ethical terms. You might not have anticipated all of the ethical debates in a subject area, but these are often best explored with the guidance of an experienced lecturer.
6. Summation	If the lecture has been successful, you are likely to have a sense of discovery by its end, but you may also be left with some discomforts or doubts. Make a note of these so that you can consult the lecturer or your personal tutor later.
7. Next direction	A successful lecture may well have added questions that you wish to answer, those beyond the opening ones which you started with.

Table 4.1 Questioning, thinking and lecture content

Listening and making notes

It is important to trust your memory as you engage with the lecture. Let me explain what I mean by that. A common student concern in lectures is to record as much information as possible because you fear that you will otherwise forget everything: 'If I could but note more information down, later I would write the perfect essay!' In practice, though, if your notes from the lecture are chock-full of quotes, facts and theories, it is likely that you may have missed many of the connecting ideas which the lecturer shared. For example, why is cancer staging so important? How does the nurse gather together information to help the patient cope with what cancer staging reveals? The questions of 'why' and 'how' are more difficult to capture when you are making real-time notes in the lecture. It requires so many more words to adequately record, and in the meantime the lecture has moved on. For that reason, it is important to polish your notes (i.e. turn them into sentences and paragraphs, fuller bullet points) after the lecture, and in the meantime listen more to what the lecturer is saying.

This raises the question of what your notes should look like as they leave the lecture room (see Activity 4.3). Because learning is also a personal matter, I do not wish to be didactic about how to take notes in a lecture. I do, however, want to recommend a basic drafting layout for the note-taking page that aids critical thinking afterwards. The trick is to capture enough notes to enable you to write a fuller summary after the lecture.

Start by dividing each blank page of your notes into three columns. If it helps, work with the pages in landscape rather than portrait format. The left-hand column should be a relatively narrow one, perhaps just 20 per cent of the page width. Label this 'lecture link'. It is simply going to be the place where you note the slide or screen that the notes relate to. Having this link to your lecture and handout will enable you to connect your thinking accurately to the points made by the lecturer. So, perhaps in this column I might record 'slide 1: role of cancer staging'. This is the title of the slide that the lecturer displayed and it is probably also the title used for the same section of the lecture handout. If you are permitted to audio-record the lecture, then it might also refer to the recording point where important points were made.

I suggest that you label the middle column of the page 'themes'. It is here that you will jot down your ideas, questions and pivotal points that seem to relate closely to the stage of the lecture that you have recorded in the left-hand column. In this area, you are going to jot down your thoughts – it is not a space to try to recreate the lecturer's slide or handout. The urge to try to reproduce all that the lecturer presents is a very human one, but try to resist it. Negotiate the supply of regular handouts and trust your notes as a place to think on paper. This column should occupy around 60 per cent of the width of your page. Perhaps here I might write things such as 'Staging indicates disease progression', 'Late stage equals disease spread/poorer prognosis', 'But staging different for different cancers', 'Wow, how to explain this to the patient?' and 'Does staging change if treatment successful?' Do you see how it comprises just snippet information and questions? It includes my emotional responses too (e.g. 'wow'). These become your prompts for fuller notes after the lecture has finished. Remember that the proportion of time spent in lectures at university is relatively small – more time should indeed be dedicated to note development.

I suggest that you label the right-hand column of the page 'keywords/references' (around 20 per cent of page width). If the lecturer does not provide a handout, then you will need a space to copy down any pivotal references that you should follow up later. You will need to explore keywords in the library to deepen your command of the ideas shared. A keyword (or phrase) in the example lecture that I am using might be 'distal spread'. This refers to the existence of tumour cells in a new area of the body, perhaps the other side of the mediastinum. Distal spread is important because it affects available treatment modalities.

Activity 4.4   Critical thinking

Look back now at your refllections in Activity 4.3 and determine whether the idea of a structured note page linked to lecture handouts helps you. Does it help you to order your notes and facilitate revision for coursework assignments or examimnations? If these notes need polishing in a subsequent write-up, how do you think this might benefit the development of your critical thinking?

I offer some of my own suggestions at the end of the chapter.

The use of questions to facilitate learning

Questions feature regularly within lectures, although many students worry about these. They fear that a question posed by the tutor will seem difficult, and that not venturing an answer or offering the wrong answer might tarnish their reputation. You will only develop your critical thinking abilities, however, if you are prepared to engage in questions, both asking your own and answering those of your tutor. Questions enable you to fill in gaps in your knowledge and ascertain whether your current grasp of a subject is complete. Tutors know that it feels daunting for a student to engage in questioning, so they use a technique that allows the more confident students to venture answers to questions first. As you attend your next lecture, notice how the tutor poses a question first to the whole group, inviting possible answers from students. The tutor 'poses' the question, then 'pauses', allowing time for everyone to give the question due consideration, and then 'pounces'. If 'pounce' sounds rather intimidating, remember that pose/pause/pounce is simply an aide-memoire for teachers learning their craft. The 'pounce' usually involves inviting a student who has signalled an interest in answering to proceed with their point. Tutors are taught *not* to embarrass individual students in the class. Where your answer is incomplete, you will usually be congratulated on the successful part of the answer before the tutor invites others to add to it: 'Gina has given us part of the answer here; who can add some more?'

Posing your own questions requires a little thought. It is important to configure a question that is comprehensible to the tutor – one to which others might also perhaps wish to hear an answer – and to ensure that this is a question, not a comment. Students frequently mix up the two, leaving the tutor unsure how best to respond, or at worst feeling that their teaching has been undermined. Here is Stewart (one of our case study nursing students) posing a very successful question associated with a lecture on cancer and altered body image:

> *I was interested in the points that you made about the sort of cancer which patients have and the effect of this on their body image. Some tumours are especially threatening. I've recently nursed a man who had a mouth cancer and he has had to have radical surgery. I wondered whether cancers that affect the face are more distressing?*

In this example, Stewart does three things. First, he orientates the tutor to where his question is focused: 'I was interested in the points that you made about …' Second, he gives the briefest rationale for posing the question: 'I've recently nursed a man …' Then he poses the question itself: 'I wondered whether …' Stewart may already have a good idea that patients with head and neck cancers suffer a higher incidence of altered body image – he has witnessed their distress. But he still manages to phrase this as a question that the tutor can answer and others can understand.

Activity 4.5   Reflection

In the next lecture that you attend, pay particular attention to the ways in which questions are posed by students. Does the quality of questioning significantly enhance what you take away from a lecture? What do you think that the student who asks questions takes away from the session that other students might not? Rather tellingly, Fatima observed to me once, 'A lecture is a performance, but it's not only that of the lecturer. Sometimes students perform too.'

As this answer is based on your own observation, there is no outline answer at the end of the chapter.

After the lecture has finished

Beyond the lecture, there remains other work to be done. Here is my 'to do' list:

- Expand on your notes in order to produce a resource that can assist you with assessments. You may need to consult a textbook to clarify your thinking at this point, or perhaps lecture notes that the teacher may have posted on the course web page. Writing points out as paragraphs forces you to express your reasoning in ways that real-time lecture notes cannot. Remember that in Chapter 3, I highlighted the value of speculation as part of higher-level critical thinking, so do not be afraid to include questions and possible ideas about what might be important, what might be happening in your notes.

- Identify any things that you do not understand. Where will you find fuller explanations? Perhaps this is something that will be available through a discussion in your personal tutor group. It is unwise to assume that a lecture will have explained everything and that you will be left query-free. Recognising what you do not yet know is part of that which drives future learning.
- Make a reflective note concerning your perceptions at this point. If you found some of the arguments made by the tutor unsettling or startling, determine why this is. What within your past experience, attitudes or values led you to alternative perspectives? What, if anything, needs to change now?

Chapter summary

Lectures are probably the learning opportunity that students think they know the most about and sometimes learn the least from. Overexposure to lectures, as well as making assumptions that one can get by frantically note-taking about everything, can undermine what can be achieved by full engagement with a lecture. Lectures are a common feature within nursing courses, so it is foolish not to derive the maximum benefit from them. By engaging with the lecture and its subject matter, you can learn a great deal and contribute to the successful learning of others. This chapter has highlighted how some preliminary questions can serve to improve your engagement with what the lecturer has to share. It has outlined how the questions that you then pose, as well as answer, materially enrich everyone's learning. Critically evaluating what the lecturer says exercises you in the sort of higher-level thinking that will be valued by assessors in your coursework later.

Preparing carefully for the lecture and following up with polished notes will significantly enhance what you learn. Materially, though, it is perhaps the quality of thinking within the lecture that determines whether you will develop the inquisitive attitudes that are so important in nursing. In the lecture, you witness the reasoning of another – the tutor.

Activities: brief outline answers

Activity 4.2 Reflection (page 74)

In this session, the visiting speaker planned to engage the students' emotional intelligence as part of learning, that which is concerned with insight and empathy into the circumstances and needs of others. She directly acquainted the student group with uncertainty and a little anxiety. In doing so, she hoped to engage the students' imaginations, helping them to picture what life could be like for patients and their relatives. It wasn't simply a 'trick'. In several subject areas (e.g. care of the dying, dealing with anxiety, rapid or radical change), feeling and expressing empathy are especially important. Coming to this session with some preconsidered questions might have been useful. For example, if you had already considered what seemed caring when patients felt uncertain, you might have engaged faster with the visiting speaker because you understood the rationale of her teaching approach.

Activity 4.4 Critical thinking (page 79)

I think three things are important when it comes to note-taking in lectures. First, from the outset, you should learn to trust your own thinking. If the course is simply perceived as an exercise in collecting information, you are much more likely to write coursework assignments that are criticised for being too descriptive. Tutors want you to think. Your notes in the lecture, then, should consist of thoughts, with the briefest prompts from what the lecture has provided. The second important thing is to connect what you think to what was taught. This is why it is good to arrange the note page in three coloumns so that you can link a handout to what you wrote down. The third thing is to successfully connect this lecture to follow-up work, perhaps some reading or a tutorial discussion. This is why the third column on the notes page is so important.

I strongly recommend expanding your lecture notes after the session has finished. Writing out fuller sentences and paragraphs reinforces the learning from the session and makes revision much easier. A handout and brief notes will seem less clear several months later. If you work consistently in this way, building a note-taking approach and writing up points afterwards, you will develop an excellent reasoning and revision aid.

Further reading

McPherson, F. (2018) *Effective Notetaking*, 3rd edition. Wellington: Wayz Press.

Fiona McPherson offers a comprehensive review of different note-taking strategies, including the use of concept analysis and spider diagrams. The argument runs that if you transform your notes into a different and perhaps more visual form, you reinforce learning and build connections to other subject matters. This is a useful book for students and tutors alike, and could also help to shape lecture designs.

Roberts, M. (2015) *Critical Thinking and Writing for Mental Health Nursing Students*. London: SAGE/Learning Matters.

I want to alert you to this companion volume from SAGE/Learning Matters for a specific reason, having recently spent time writing and reviewing within the field of mental healthcare. Mental healthcare has a continuing debate about the nature of health, wellness and illness, as well as about what constitute the best therapies to help patients. Attending lectures in this field, then, is likely to expose you to a series of arguments and counterarguments, a range of theories perhaps more divergent than in other areas of practice. I think that it will seem a useful read as you make sense of the cases made to you, as well as helping to develop the sort of professional empathetic attitudes that are important to patient care.

Useful websites

www.lucidchart.com/blog/weaving-ideas-with-spider-diagrams

Spider diagrams are an excellent way to polish and rework notes that you have made during a lecture. They are especially well-suited to visually indicating factors that contribute to a problem or need, or perhaps connections, causes and effects associated with illness or treatment. Some students also use them within their lecture notes, but I recommend them instead for revision work, when you reduce complex information to essentials for answers in an examination. Lauren McNeely's explanation of the spider diagram here is simple and should enable you to develop your own diagrams very quickly indeed.

www.youtube.com/watch?v=Y9LBUf1NzU0

As the speaker in this video on how to improve your listening skills suggests, we all think we know how to listen effectively, but he makes a persuasive case that this is not always the case. It is well worth reviewing the video to improve your chances of securing the most from the nursing lectures that you attend. Do not worry that the examples do not come from nursing – the principles still apply.

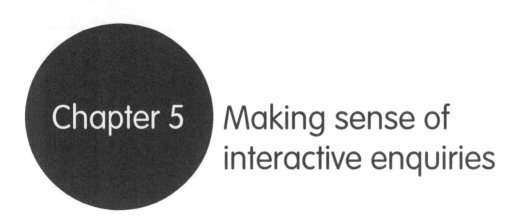

Chapter 5 — Making sense of interactive enquiries

Chapter aims

After reading this chapter, you will be able to:

- describe the key features of interactive enquiry;
- indicate how you need to prepare for and attend to the different learning opportunities offered there;
- contrast learning in these settings with that in the lecture.

Introduction

Your nursing studies are broadly arranged using three types of learning activity. The most traditionally associated with university is the lecture, although healthcare courses are increasingly diversifying the learning you are asked to participate in. Skill labs, for instance, provide demonstrations with 'you try now' opportunities to follow. The second learning activity is that associated with interactive enquiries, which in this book includes the work you share with others in **seminars**, workshops and role play. Chapter 7 deals with online learning, which is also clearly interactive. The third type of learning activity is that conducted within clinical areas, within the different placements associated with your course.

Each of the different learning activities assist you to develop the sorts of insight, knowledge and practice template thinking that you will need to be a successful nurse. Historically, lectures have majored in delivering large amounts of information, the 'what' of nursing care. As well as learning about the 'what' of care, though, you need to learn about the 'why' of care: Why do we approach patients this way? Why is it important to understand the patient's beliefs and perspectives? Interactive enquiries are especially suited to this area of learning activity (Koivisto et al., 2016; K.-C. Lee et al., 2018). It exercises you in deliberations that do not always offer a definitively correct way to proceed. We need to weigh up the merits of handling care in particular ways, which is best understood when we talk about the process of care, draw on the experience of others, and check and balance our beliefs about what might work well. Research does not necessarily guide us on how to arrange care effectively and efficiently. We need to anticipate practicum, a learned way of arranging care that expresses best principles and acknowledges service resources and constraints (Kaihlanen et al., 2018). So, the 'how' of nursing care is also explored through interactive enquiry (J.J. Lee et al., 2018).

Interactive enquiries serve a very important role as you work towards forming the templates for nursing care. They help you to develop the ability to make a case of your own and conduct debates (Gambrill and Gibbs, 2017). These forms of learning activity permit no hiding place from the responsibility to decide some things for yourself. In clinical practice, care is negotiated and consulted upon. You will have to express professional values and argue for what seems to be the best care. There is no standard text to tell you what is right. That sounds pretty daunting, I know; but if the learning sessions are well-run, then there is no reason why this should not be the most fruitful of learning activities.

So, what characterises interactive enquiries?

- You are usually provided with relatively modest resources to set you off (briefing materials).
- You will need to liaise with your fellow students. A tutor or librarian will guide you, but they will not tell you what to think.
- You will need to structure your enquiries, the information gathering, sifting and sorting, and that which is discovered. This will often involve work in the library or on the internet.
- You will need to communicate in a collegiate way. That means listening attentively to others, respecting expertise where available, and accepting that not all lines of enquiry will necessarily provide the answers that you hoped for.

Gina had the following to say about this sort of learning activity:

I found the interactive group learning pretty difficult at first. I think that was down to two things. First, it seemed to require so much more effort! Tutors were acquainting us with the insecurity of practice reasoning in as safe a way as they could. The second reason it seemed tough was that the group work required me to trust other students and what they knew. I didn't know for sure that they could teach me much. I had to learn to trust them and to discover that some colleagues were particularly good at some things – for instance, interpreting research reports.

Activity 5.1   Reflection

Have you felt the same way as Gina about interactive enquiries? Later Gina said that she felt her points were a confession of laziness. I explained that much past elementary study was descriptive – you simply became aware of ideas, issues and facts, but did not question them. In past studies, you did not have to take responsibility for evaluating or using them. Nursing required a shift to the latter, and that was unnerving. Interactive group learning is about developing enquiry resilience. You need to believe that you can understand and solve problems.

Reflect on this with a chosen colleague. Sometimes acknowledging that you each have fears can serve to build courage.

As this answer is based on your own observation, there is no outline answer at the end of the chapter.

Learning from role play

Fatima told me that she hates role-play learning. She was quite emphatic about the matter: 'If I wanted to act, I would have gone to drama school!' Her anxiety is entirely normal. When role-playing, you risk discovering things about how you think at exactly the same time as they are exhibited to the others involved. By role play, I mean a carefully orchestrated and time-limited interaction of a group of students (and sometimes others), each of whom has a defined role to play while exploring a process, circumstance, opportunity or problem that is relevant in nursing. The role play includes a briefing (sometimes you are asked to research your role in the library first), a period of interaction where you enter the role and imagine how care might seem, and then afterwards a period of debrief where you take stock of the experience (Presti, 2019). To make role play feel more accessible, it is important to acknowledge that you are trying out ideas, interactions, ways to express care. Role play might help you to uncover some deeply held attitudes, values and beliefs; if it does, your tutor will help you to examine those in the most supportive way possible – Aydin Er et al. (2017) detail just how important nursing values are to students in nursing. Your tutor will encourage fellow students to reflect on the episode with you, about your role, in a constructive and encouraging way.

In role play, the tutor remains attentive, ready to call a time out so that you can share a conversation about any issues that arise. Sometimes you may be asked to be the observer of a colleague's role play, providing them with thoughtful feedback. A skilful tutor will allow the role play to develop for several minutes and will then help you to pick out some observations about what was happening. Key points might attend to:

* whether the activity was proceeding as anticipated (why or why not?);
* whether you felt comfortable with what you were doing or saying;
* whether you felt that you understood what another person did or said;
* whether there are other ways in which you could have handled a particular interaction.

Table 5.1 details some critical thinking benefits of role-play learning that I think you should consider.

Role-play feature	Critical thinking benefit
Imagining yourself in the role of another (e.g. a distressed relative)	We rarely have the opportunity to imagine the experiences, perceptions and approaches of others. In role play, you exercise your imagination to understand how contexts help to shape interactions, something that you have read about as a higher-order feature of reasoning in Chapter 1.
Focusing upon professionally relevant interactions	It is very difficult for theory to seem practice-authentic. Learning on campus seems to operate in a rarefied and privileged place. Role-play focuses on relatively discrete interactions that enable us to anticipate how care in action might seem. Seeing what is realistically possible teaches us about what nurses focus upon, how they negotiate care.
Exploring beliefs and values, those you imagine others might use	Beliefs and values shape a great deal in healthcare, although they are not necessarily analysed in everyday clinical conversations. Role-playing situations of tension or conflict can help us to analyse how we and others approach the world around us. Because we acted 'in role' with support, we can then review the insights gained.
Exercising safe decisions about what to do next	In Part 1, I emphasised the importance of developing templates, ways in which nurses enact care, weighing up what is realistic. It would seem daunting to have to do that again and again in practice from scratch. In role play, we can try out solutions and examine what seemed to work best.
Reacting in real time to how others behave	In Chapter 2, we briefly explored why reflection in action is more difficult. Hindsight helps us to improve upon our reasoning. Role play, with its debrief, provides both forms of reflective activity.

(Continued)

Table 5.1 (Continued)

Role-play feature	Critical thinking benefit
Comparing experience with research/teaching/theory	Nursing information, ideas and plans need to be realistic. In role play, you have the chance to try out what it takes to express a theory, to use teaching or research findings.
Exploring the emotional labour of practice	Nursing work can seem draining as we have to demonstrate emotional intelligence, working with the needs and perspectives of others. Understanding what may seem most tiring is important if you are to think and act strategically.

Table 5.1 Features of role play and critical thinking benefits

I asked Fatima and Raymet what they found helped them to prepare for role play. Below is what they told me – I have also annotated each response with reflections of my own.

Fatima

I need quite a lot of reassurance about role play, especially if there is a new tutor leading the session. For that reason, I make a point of checking with the tutor beforehand what the purpose of the role play is.

It is important that the tutor sets out the purpose and the planned process for role-play learning sessions. I sometimes say to students that they are not yet qualified nurses, so this is a form of pretend play, much as happens in childhood. Here, we can try out ideas, positions and perspectives. Even if they have to be modified to be acceptable, we can do that in a very supportive way. The role play is a learning activity, not an assessment. You cannot fail it, but you might need to do some extra thinking based on insights gained. You are allowed to signal when explorations seem too much or you need a break.

Raymet

I've found that how well I do in role-play sessions depends on how stressed I am before the session, whether I perhaps feel tense about something else entirely. Then I say to myself, 'This is play time.' The easiest role plays for me are where the roles, the situations, are entirely new to me. Then I don't have baggage to expose, at least any that I'm aware of.

Notice Raymet's concern about role play as a performance – she wants to act well. Role play, though, is simply a vehicle for learning and it will require some focused imaginative work. You need to be sincere in imagining what the role entails. Raymet makes an excellent point about fresh situations. If we role-play there, our 'performance' might be less polished, but there seems to be less risk that we will reveal something which we have doubts about. My recommendation is to write up reflections on the role play, including your feelings and insights, after the session has ended.

Activity 5.2   Critical thinking

Jot down now some practice situations that you think it would be good to explore in class using role play.

Discuss these with your fellow students to see if you have common needs. Consider asking your module tutor to see if selected role plays could then be arranged.

As this answer is based on your own observation, there is no outline answer at the end of the chapter.

Learning within seminars

Interaction is also equally important in seminars, another form of group learning. In a seminar, individual students are briefed to fulfil different information-gathering tasks within the literature or on the internet, and to bring back their discoveries to the group, sharing what they have found and discussing what this might mean with their fellow students (Morgan, 2019). Seminars are typically arranged within a tutorial group, where no more than 10–12 students make a contribution.

Seminars are designed to teach you study skills (especially those relating to search and find), project management skills (you need to work to a common project end) and critical thinking skills (a weighing up of evidence and options available). You will need to be disciplined in your work and brave enough to report your discoveries. Because everyone is asked to contribute in this way, seminars also teach you that you can learn from fellow students as well as your tutor.

Activity 5.3   Group work

As it takes a little while to build confidence as a seminar learner, you might find it useful to practise this work informally with some of your fellow students before you tackle a bigger exercise within a class. Choose a healthcare news story reported in the press. Next, each take a different newspaper that reports the story and summarise what is focused upon, how the issue is portrayed. Then report your findings back to an informal student group to gain an understanding of how stories may vary. Did all of the newspapers identify the same issues? This is what a seminar involves – the gathering and critical comparison of information.

As this answer is based on your own observation, there is no outline answer at the end of the chapter.

During the search stage of any seminar work, you will need to find the best possible paper or website information to share. If you bring back something that is not quite clear, more discussion work will be needed at the end. During the report and discussion stage of the seminar, it is important to present a clear summary of your discovery and what you make of it. Afterwards, you will need to stand ready with constructive questions for those who present their work (e.g. 'How confident do you feel about the author's claims?').

Seminar work challenges you to: discriminate (e.g. about what material to use); interpret (e.g. about what authors really argue); speculate (e.g. regarding what might be the significance of evidence uncovered); and make arguments (e.g. regarding what care now seems justified). Your tutor is likely to work within the seminar group to help you do a number of things:

- determine that what you seem to be concluding, or what you agree for the time being, remains uncertain (summarising);
- explore other questions and consider alternative perspectives;
- identify when your discussions are going 'off-track' – the tutor's contributions, though, will often remain speculative in nature and they will be at pains not to instruct you.

Stewart and I discussed his approach to preparing for seminar work. It may give you confidence to learn that Stewart consistently achieved A or B grades in his coursework, with tutors highlighting his ability to successfully organise information. I have listed his commendable suggestions:

1. Do not prevaricate – searching for information takes more time than you might imagine.
2. Ask the tutor to clarify the focus of the seminar before you proceed to search for information. Some of the best seminars are arranged in terms of answers to a set question.
3. Collaborate quickly and regularly. Sometimes you will work alone to bring information back to a seminar, but quite often the search work is shared. If so, check that you have the means to contact one another – that way you can minimise the risk that information is missed or duplicated.
4. Make meticulous notes as regards the source material. It is frustrating to try to locate work with inadequate references later.
5. Jot down your questions as you read. Do this immediately after you have read a piece of literature.
6. Do not be afraid to acknowledge gaps in your knowledge after your search work is completed. Other students may bring back information that fills in a gap for you. In any case, some areas of healthcare have a patchy evidence base.

Learning within workshops

Among the workshops that you might be invited to take part in are the following:

- *Masterclasses:* An expert practitioner helps you to rehearse your practice skills (Hingston and Cross, 2017). Masterclasses combine demonstration with guidance and feedback as you attempt to emulate practice (e.g. listening techniques to assist anxious patients).
- *Problem-based learning sessions:* These are typically based on patient care scenarios (Compton et al., 2020). You and your colleagues are invited to use available evidence to work out what the important issues are, what is problematic, and how you will then proceed (e.g. managing a patient's chronic pain).

What often distinguishes a workshop from a seminar is that it centres on how to combine different elements of care, wedding evidence, information and skills review together, for example. While the seminar classically emphasises reading within the literature, a workshop might ask you to interview practitioners on their care strategies, perhaps requiring you to review healthcare policies and link them to recent research. A workshop often operates more closely to the sort of template thinking that you first read about in Chapter 1. Gina especially liked workshop learning. She noted:

Nursing is untidy, work never complete, and workshop learning assures me that others see it that way too. I used to think that others had perfect and complete answers – they don't!

Activity 5.4   Reflection

Here are two areas where I have helped students within a workshop approach. Each required the marrying of information, skills and practice context insights. On each occasion, I worked with one or more clinicians to enhance the learning opportunities for students. Why do you think each was especially suited to a workshop approach?

1. Helping patients to come to terms with having a permanent colostomy after surgery for bowel cancer.

2. Helping patients to make sense of their anxiety disorder.

An outline answer is given at the end of this chapter.

Gina and I agree that workshop learning works best when three things happen. First, there is a sense of achievement linked to the discoveries made, both personal and those that the group managed between them. So, begin by expecting to discover something personally important that you can share. Second, there is surprise at what is discovered through group work (about the subject but also collective endeavour). Third, there is pleasure in working with others within a group that seems to 'gel'. Nursing emphasises teamwork and collaboration, as well as learning from experience, so workshops are an important way of learning. The ability to develop and then demonstrate independent thought, right at the top of the critical thinking and reflective reasoning hierarchy, is closely associated with a willingness to collaborate towards shared discoveries.

Managing uncertainty

At the heart of all interactive enquiry is the need to manage uncertainty. What is required of us, of me, and what shall we do to manage the project set before us? What might be achieved, missed or perhaps misunderstood? What mistakes might happen to confuse our understanding of a subject? If we can manage uncertainty, learning becomes more pleasurable.

If interactive enquiry left no uncertainty, no issues to debate, there would be no scope for learning through experience. We would not understand what effort it takes to reach decisions or to make policies or protocols, and we would not understand how groups can operate together to develop strategies of their own. Fatima felt the uncertainty of her interactive enquiry learning activities acutely. She observed:

> *What alarmed me was not only just how much we didn't know, but how unsettling it was then to agree on the best ways to act. I craved assurance and only gradually learned to trust our group to make good decisions.*

Activity 5.5   Critical thinking

Look at the following list of possible ways of resolving interactive learning uncertainty and decide which of these could have helped you with past problems. That experience may come from a past course or even outside of nursing – the principles still hold good.

- Ask the tutor/group advisor to clarify the project or learning brief before you set off.
- Check what arrangements are in place for ensuring that work proceeds in the right direction.
- Set out a schedule of work, agreeing what sorts of activities are needed and deciding in what order these will be tackled.
- Agree a means of recording your progress, the decisions agreed, and the discoveries made.

- Determine group etiquette (i.e. an agreed way of talking about each other's contributions).

As this answer is based on your own observation, there is no outline answer at the end of the chapter.

To complete your interactive enquiry activities, it is necessary to start with the clearest possible brief. If yours seems unclear, you should ask your tutor to clarify points for you. In most instances, group activities are supported by a written brief. Within a problem-based learning exercise, for example, there is likely to be one or more patient case studies and associated tasks to complete (Compton et al., 2020). Typically, too, the project will set out the aims and objectives of the exercise so that you can sense what work is necessary.

While tutors do not direct the work of the group, they are required to monitor your work. It is a good idea, then, to check with the tutor when they will intervene to ensure that enquiries continue in an appropriate way. Consulting with the tutor on a regular basis in projects that span several weeks is important.

Project groups are usually composed of people with a mix of aptitudes, and it is certainly not expected that all group members will be good at everything. Indeed, sometimes the tutor devises project groups to help students explore and share their aptitudes. To gain the benefit, however, you will need to be prepared to volunteer what you feel comfortable doing, even if you believe your work might not be perfect. You will also need to acknowledge the work done by others who have other talents. Setting aside personal insecurities is part of the learning process. Start with the assumption that we all have insecurities, many of which are unspoken. What is more important now is that what you share works to achieve project ends.

Wasted time increases the pressures on a group, especially as they near the point where they must present their findings. For that reason, agreeing a schedule of work, as well as how much time is allocated to each part of the project, helps to discipline the enquiry.

Instead of a project that finishes with a lot of information about just one thing, you will have a project that seems balanced and measured, professional and insightful. It is then necessary to keep a brief record of the lines of enquiry and the decisions made. Such an 'audit trail' enables the group to tell the story of their enquiry, as well as presenting the end product of what they have learned.

Simple group etiquette rules ensure that colleagues are treated with respect and that each contributes in an adequate measure to the work in hand. For example, rules might set out expectations regarding attending meetings, supplying copies of interesting evidence found, and listening attentively until a colleague has presented the whole of their findings. Most project briefs will refer to such group etiquette and set some working parameters.

Chapter summary

Interactive enquiry activities represent some of the most active learning that you are likely to engage in. Interactive learning is proactive, challenging you to engage with project challenges, contributing questions and solutions as you proceed. While they require significant personal effort and imagination, they have the benefit of bridging the gap between theory and practice. Role play, for example, simulates the untidiness of clinical conversation. If you elect to conduct role plays on concerns that have arisen while on clinical placements, you will find that they quickly become engaging.

Seminars and workshops emphasise learning within the group. You will learn as much about the process and enquiry as about the subject matter of the project work shared. You will need to be well organised here, diligent and consultative. Reasoning in these contexts requires more collaboration and effort. It is an investment well made, however. Much of the nursing you will practise later relies upon just such shared learning.

Activities: brief outline answers

Activity 5.4 Reflection (page 91)

Helping patients to come to terms with having a permanent colostomy after surgery for bowel cancer

The workshop approach was especially useful in this instance because my clinical colleague offered brief illustrations of how she talked about stomas to patients, and I added some theory on changes to body image caused by the diagnosis of bowel cancer. We then invited the students to select questions that patients had asked about their colostomy from a hat, and invited the group to discuss the best ways to answer these.

Helping patients to make sense of their anxiety disorder

In this workshop, the students first generated ideas about admission to hospital that they believed would worry patients with a pre-existing anxiety disorder. A clinical psychologist then explored with the students how they had selected their ideas and why they believed these particular aspects of hospital admission might cause alarm. I acted as secretary to the group, recording the conclusions reached, and then related that to the theory of risk assessment.

Further reading

If you are engaged in running role-play activities as a nurse, the following textbooks will be valuable. Both assume some familiarity with education, but the principles of how best to proceed are still clearly set out.

Heinrich, P. (2017) *When Role Play Comes Alive: A Theory and Practice.* London: Palgrave Macmillan.

Paul Heinrich is an unashamed advocate of role play in healthcare, and I share that enthusiasm. There is considerable scope to use role play to enhance the compassion base of nurse education.

Oriot, D. and Alinier, G. (2018) *Pocket Book for Simulation Debriefing in Healthcare.* London: Springer.

One of the arguments made by Heinrich (above) is that for role play to be effective, individuals have to engage in it wholeheartedly. Like actors, we must feel our way into the part played, imagining how the character feels. This offers great rewards and insights, but it also requires some skillful debriefing. The tutor needs to help the nurse step back outside the exercise and re-examine what has been discovered. Sometimes that involves reviewing some painful experiences. This book, then, seems the logical complement to the above text for anyone planning to lead simulation/role play.

Useful websites

www.prepareforsuccess.org.uk/taking_part_in_seminars.php

This short podcast from Southampton University is aimed at overseas students less familiar with seminar learning. It is, though, a good summary for all, emphasising the importance of preparation for the seminar and active involvement within it.

www.youtube.com/watch?v=cMtLXXf9Sko

This is a cogent summary of the main elements of problem-based learning from Maastricht University, and how this commonly fits into a wider curriculum. Many universities incorporate elements of problem-based learning into nursing tutorial work. Notice the emphasis on roles within the problem-solving group and how the tutor works to assist you with any impasses that can arise.

Chapter 6　Making clinical placements successful

Chapter aims

After reading this chapter, you will be able to:

*   summarise the nature of critical enquiry that you need to engage in within clini-cal placements;

- detail what preparations will enable you to complete a successful clinical placement;
- discuss the part played by the student–practice supervisor relationship in a satisfying and effective learning placement;
- understand the reflective and open approach you must use if feedback is to aid your studies.

Introduction

Your clinical placements are a vital part of course study and typically account for about half of all the learning that you will complete. Going on placement, though, is an important learning transition and one that has not always been well explained. Yes, there may be a series of clinical placement objectives, but these have often focused on subject areas such as cancer treatment rather than your personal needs, linked perhaps to clinical resoning and skills. This is the 'what' of learning, areas of module subject matter that we hope clinical learning will reinforce. The really valuable clinical learning extends well beyond the 'what' of nursing, into the 'why' and the 'how' of practice (Higgs et al., 2019). The fundamental purpose of learning in clinical practice is to learn the successful templates of clinical reasoning that you read about in Chapter 1. This will include elements of professional etiquette, rules and regulations, but it will also examine how best to do the right thing at the right time (Hutchinson et al., 2017).

What has compounded the placement learning challenge is that some practice supervisors have struggled to allocate time and clear explanation to learners in clinical settings (Sundler et al., 2019). It has been tempting to hope that students will 'pick things up as they go along'. Sometimes that happens, but in my experience relying on a learning knack in new environments is not ideal. It is better to approach the clinical learning environment with a clear critical thinking perspective in hand. You need to identify learning opportunities to recognise successful care, as well as writing up experiences using a reflective practice model.

If you are to discover the sorts of templates referred to in Chapter 1, you will need to engage in some pattern recognition. Do not worry – you are already very good at it. Your brain has developed to notice what seems to fit with what (Smith et al., 2015). Human beings are predisposed to search for events that emerge in some sort of a coherent way, to look for order in chaos. However, because clinical environments offer a significant amount of stimuli, experiences that you can attend to, there is merit in asking you to work in a slightly more focused way. Instead of trying to practise all the reasoning attributes you read about in Chapter 1, it is better to instead start with just a few questions.

In Chapter 4, I encouraged you to approach lectures using a short series of questions, those about context, connections (or correlations), causes and consequences, and caring. Similar questions will serve you very well in practice placements too, as well as being of assistance to practice supervisors who wish to help develop your thinking. In Table 6.1, I indicate how they can help both you and your practice supervisor. As Sue (our case study registered nurse) also acts as a practice supervisor for students on her ward, she has illustrated the explanations from a supervision perspective.

Context	Explanations
What is the context for the event(s) that I am witnessing?	Your selection of interesting events relates to your current module of study and perceived learning needs (see Chapter 2), but beyond that the focusing of your attention usefully begins with the context of the episode witnessed. For example, was this a new patient to the ward (new patients perhaps have common needs)? Was the patient improving or deteriorating? In pattern recognition, the context is like a backdrop – it is that against which everything else is registered. Context helps explain what seems noteworthy. *Sue: Contexts seem very familiar to me, but some still surprise me, and I'm likely to point them out as learning opportunities for students. I want my student to understand why I have had to 'think again'.*
Connections or correlations What seems to fit with that observed? (If you prefer, what usually seems to happen alongside it?)	We rarely notice a single act or speech. We notice a small collection of acts or words, action and interaction. This is what makes the care episode. It is what becomes a viable focus for a reflective practice model. But we still need to make sense of the different elements, how they fit together. Some elements might seem unusual, or perhaps missing, and this prompts curiosity or unease as we witness events – something seems odd. *Sue: I remember a patient who had recently been diagnosed with lung cancer. He seemed especially concerned about viral infections. What wasn't clear at first was whether he realised that cancer and its treatment made him more prone to infections or whether he wondered if cancer was caused by an infection. Understanding how he thought was important!*
Causes and consequences What appears to bring the event about and what can seem to follow on from it?	Your business in practice is often to do with investigating origins of problems, anticipating and countering consequences. So, patterns have a before and an after, often a cause and an effect. Skilful nurses read events and needs that way – it is part of their template thinking. *Sue: My student and I asked the patient whether he thought you could catch cancer. He said yes, in a way you could. So, we started to ask about how he thought that happened, and he referred to human papillomavirus and the risk of cervical cancer. He had read about that. He reasoned that chest infections probably did the same sort of damage to lungs. We started to understand that he didn't exactly think cancer was a virus, but that a sufficient viral load could trigger cancer development. The origin of cancer for him was to do with viral load and the frequency of chest infections.* What Sue and her student are learning about is the patient's narrative, his explanation of events and what he believes about his illness. To individualise care, we need to hear and understand the patient's narrative (Price, 2019b).

Context	Explanations
Caring What about this event or episode exemplifies caring, or conversely that which is uncaring?	Once you have started to attend to the pattern in terms of context, connections, and causes and effects, there is a need to act in some way. In nursing, this is expressed as care. Care is about comfort, psychological support, assurance and companionship, as well as treatments of different kinds.
	Sue: I asked the student what she thought we should do. She answered that we should correct the man's misunderstanding as it was causing him a lot of anxiety. Yes, we would have to warn about the infection risks associated with chemotherapy, but we shouldn't leave him feeling that he had caused his cancer through exposing himself to too many past infections. He had to live with the fact that lung cancer arose for many reasons, genetic and related to cigarette smoking.

Table 6.1   Using questions to read clinical practice

Activity 6.1   Reflection

Study Table 6.1 in order to better understand what a pattern looks like and how Sue's nursing template (personalised care) develops out of a context and an insight into the patient's narrative of illness. There was something about this patient that suggested an individual need. It arose because she saw how different bits of information seemed to be fitting together, which became important as we consider cause and effect. She and her student could support the patient better if they investigated and corrected some ideas about viruses and cancer.

As this answer is based on your own observation, there is no outline answer at the end of the chapter.

Building a clinical case study

The above 'C' questions work well when they focus upon clinical episodes of care, but they are even more powerful if you arrange to follow one or more case study patients for longer periods of time during your clinical placement. Nursing care is not delivered through fragmented care episodes; it is arranged as part of the care relationship. To understand that fully, there is merit in studying an individual patient's changing needs over time. Historically, such profile studies of patients and their needs led to the writing up of 'nursing care studies'. These were typically discussed with regard to a particular model of nursing. Today, case studies are being written for new purposes, such as to better explore a recurring patient problem, a nursing skill in action, or what it means to deliver person-centred care (Price, 2019b).

As you think about the 'C' questions to help frame your clinical placement enquiries, it is worth debating whether a clinical case study might assist your learning. In Chapter 11,

I detail how to write up such a clinical case study, but here I start with the characteristics of the ideal case study patient to work with. Here is what is important:

- Case study learning must be sanctioned by your practice supervisor and fit with the requirements of your module of study. The purpose of the case study is usually to illuminate patient-distinctive needs and the ways in which nurses liaise to ensure that care seems individualised.
- You must ask the patient's permission to focus enquiries on their needs and care. You are not acting as a researcher here, but rather a practitioner who focuses your reflection upon their requirements. Study will require that you ask the patient more about their experiences, what they expect of care, and how they try to liaise with the nurses and doctors. It is necessary to acquaint them with any particular focus of interest that you have. For example, perhaps the patient is coming to terms with a chronic illness, so you are especially interested in their learning about treatment and how best to cope.
- The partner patient should be someone who feels comfortable discussing their circumstances and work with care staff to address their needs. To this end, the ideal patient is probably inquisitive about their care and they feel able to articulate their experiences. Targeted reflection is not interrogation work, but the patient needs to feel assured that you will curtail the enquiries if that is what they wish.
- The patient needs to remain in your care sufficiently long to better explore needs and care negotiation. Someone admitted for day care surgery, for example, might not be such a successful subject for reflection.
- The patient should be someone that your practice supervisor also cares for. While you deliver a percentage of their care, it is important that you are also able to access how the patient and the registered nurse interact.

Your clinical placement thereafter involves regular discussions with the patient and your practice supervisor to better understand how care evolves, as well as how needs are identified and addressed. In particular, it is valuable to understand how each explains (narrates) the care in progress. Do they use the same language, for instance?

How are care plans negotiated and what does the patient know and contribute to the planning process? Your note-taking will incrementally accumulate during the course of your placement. It should include:

- Questions and reflections about what you witness. Some of the notes will constitute full reflective practice episodes, but do not be afraid to jot down passing impressions as well.
- Queries about clinical reasoning, that which your practice supervisor might explain about problem-solving.
- Summary of any related reading that you do associated with your chosen case study, which may include protocols and policies or research evidence in use.
- Periodic summaries of what you think you have discovered, which might entail detailing the order of teaching offered to a patient with a chronic illness, reviewing

what the patient mastered quickly or struggled to understand, and exploring what the patient wanted to know compared with what seemed clinically necessary to teach.

Preparing for the placement

Preparation for your placement can significantly reduce anxieties, such as those about a busy work environment and the risk of making errors there. The more you can bring order to the learning experience, working with your practice supervisor, the more constructive the learning will seem. Table 6.2 suggests what might be done in advance of your placement.

Strategy	Benefit
Review the learning outcomes that have to be achieved during this placement and any assessment arrangements that apply. Tell your supervisor about the above 'C' questions that help you to explore practice.	You focus on what has to be achieved. Practice supervisors want to show you a lot, but it can seem rather random. If you can help them to link enquiries to context, connections, causes and consequences, and care, enquiry will seem more coherent.
Research the work of the department, ward or practice by looking at any details on healthcare agency websites.	By doing some homework, you will not have to ask quite so many questions on your placement.
Revisit your portfolio to identify particular practice skills that you wish to improve on (e.g. patient history-taking).	You calmly determine what needs your attention.
Make personal contact with the clinical team, writing to or emailing the nurse in charge.	You establish an immediate rapport if you show such personal organisation.
Try to establish in advance who your practice supervisor will be.	Knowing this will increase your confidence.
Ascertain what sorts of illness, injury or other health challenges tax patients in the placement area.	The patients on a ward often share a common context, as well as similar diagnoses and needs. This might assist you to identify possible clinical case study opportunities.
Check when your first shift is and arrive in good time, correctly attired.	

Table 6.2 Getting ready for clinical placement study

Activity 6.2 Critical thinking

Imagine that you are meeting your practice supervisor for the very first time. You explain, 'I'm hoping to observe practice using some questions while I'm here, to understand care as you do. Can I explain the questions to you?' The practice supervisor says, 'Yes, of course!' So, how will you explain context, connections, causes and consequences, and care with regard to pattern recognition and template thinking?

Some suggestions are given at the end of this chapter.

Chapter 6

Working with your practice supervisor

Students are not always aware of what a supervisor brings to student support, so let us summarise that. Practice supervisors are experienced practitioners who are familiar with their area of care and its local policies and protocols. They have undertaken a short course in the principles of learning, teaching, support and assessment, and they are charged with guiding you during your clinical placement. They act as advocates of learning, but they also have responsibilities to inculcate you into the team and its work (Bifarin and Stonehouse, 2017). They work to help you master skills and apply your knowledge, but retain responsibilities towards their patients, colleagues and the profession. Practice supervisors share unique insights into the practical ways of conducting nursing work (Ryan and McAllister, 2020).

Successful work with your practice supervisor will:

- help you to manage your anxieties about learning in the clinical setting;
- help you to develop an acceptable approach to enquiry in this setting;
- open doors to other expertise in the clinical setting;
- give you thoughtful and honest weekly feedback so that you are well prepared for assessments and end of placement reports;
- help you to address your own learning agenda, as well as that required by the course.

The working relationship with your practice supervisor should be one of trust and mutual respect. Practice supervisors expect students to arrive ready and eager to learn. Judging how much learning to take on, as well as how fast, in a clinical context will need to be negotiated. It will be necessary to be honest with your practice supervisor as regards what you feel you can cope with. Some learning within placement will be opportunistic. If you engage in that learning, though, request a review discussion afterwards so that you can evaluate that which was witnessed. Other learning will be skills-focused, and your practice supervisor will quite probably demonstrate several procedures – do not be afraid to ask about those afterwards.

Other learning opportunities within the clinical area may be planned rather than opportunistic. Sue, for instance, describes how she briefs her students on those:

> I have eight or nine recurring learning opportunities that I want all students to study while they are on the ward, and I've explained my thinking about that to the other clinicians. For example, we have an office round, reviewing some key patients and their treatment, before we go and talk to them at their bedsides. I want the learner to listen to what is discussed but also to consider why we proceed in that way.

Sometimes the insights gained acquaint you with difficult decisions relating to care priorities and resource allocation. Care has an etiquette dimension, one that enables professionals to work together. Your practice supervisor should take the opportunity to debrief you on these afterwards. In the above example, Sue explains that many students ask about practice as a 'managed performance'. The discussions with the patients at their bedsides are influenced by what is discussed in the office beforehand.

Working with a practice supervisor, then is not just about the best enquiry, pattern recognition and template understanding. It is not simply about skill demonstrations either. A skilful practice supervisor will help you to understand the nature of work done in the area, the ways in which the team communicate and how service is conceived. At times, this may raise ethical or logistical issues that seem startling, and these also deserve discussion with the practice supervisor. Sue observed:

> *When I first started looking after students, I worried that care had to look perfect. I believed that it had to be textbook fashion. Of course, that was impossible. Care episodes are shaped by patient requests and behaviour, as well as the resources available to care for them. At the end of a shift, patients, relatives and clinicians, all decide whether it has been a 'good day'. At best, each of the stakeholders agree what 'good' means. Even when they don't, however, the key elements of respect and concern for others must always be apparent.*

Activity 6.3   Reflection

One of the stresses associated with clinical placement learning is associated with the theory–practice gap. You might observe that not all theory can be operationalised, made to work in practice. Conversely, you might feel that clinicians are always working so hard that they struggle to exemplify the highly individual and attentive care which others have suggested is desirable. This is called a cognitive dissonance problem, where 'should' and 'could' are not the same.

Take a moment to jot down some of the dissonance issues that worry you the most and share these with your practice supervisor or personal tutor. If you cannot make 'should' and 'could' always meet in the middle, how might you judge whether your own care seems professional, satisfying and reasonable at the end of the day?

An outline answer is given at the end of this chapter.

Managing assessment

At the end of your placement, a practice assessor (one of the staff) will write up a report on your learning there. Reports cover matters such as the development of your skills, the attitudes that you demonstrate in practice, your commitment to nursing care and the gains made in your knowledge (Feeney and Everett, 2020). Today, assessment is said to be 'continuous', and we need to consider the psychology of this process, which can seem daunting.

There does need to be judgement on performance, and this remains an issue for qualified nurses. Annual staff appraisals, complaints by patients, and reviews by auditors are all part of professional life (NMC, 2019). Assessments that are made of your performance are mediated by an understanding of your stage of training and the learning objectives set. Importantly, good assessment takes account of your readiness to critically examine your own work. Insight is important, as well as practice performance (Canniford and Fox-Young, 2015). The staff are interested in your learning and your response to guidance. While you might demonstrate shortfalls in skill or knowledge, these can sometimes be compensated for by a willingness to receive instruction.

To help you manage assessment, you need to be critical of your own performance. You will need to recognise misconceptions that are not serving you well. Such a personal audit of week-by-week performance will then enable you to seek the guidance of your supervisor, and at the earliest possible point to start correcting any shortfalls and building on your successes. The following represent a series of week-by-week questions that might help you to evaluate your progress:

- What do you think was the best of my work this week and what still needed improvement?
- If you were to suggest one focus for improving my practice next week, what would it be and why?
- How do you think it feels for a patient to be nursed by me?

Assessments of your performance during a clinical placement will focus on your skills, the way in which you apply your knowledge, and your attitudes and values (Vae et al., 2018). The judgement of skills is usually well received by student nurses. Students understand that the practice supervisor and others who contribute to the assessment of your performance are skilful. Receiving critique of your applied knowledge is also usually well received, at least where the supervisor and others have asked you pertinent questions. It seems fair to critique applied knowledge where you have had the opportunity to reason aloud and demonstrate why you proceed as you do. Assessment of attitudes and values, however, can be contentious, and it sometimes feels hurtful. This is because your attitudes and values are inferred from what you do, what you say, and how you approach care and colleague relationships. When students struggle in this area of their learning, skilful coaching may need to follow.

Pause to reflect on how different the campus and the clinical environment are as places of learning. The robust enquiry and debate attitude that is so important on campus might seem aggressive in practice. Absolute thinking, something that we equated in Chapter 3 with lower levels of critical thinking and reflection, may in practice become a stereotype applied to patients or professional colleagues. It is vital that nurses learn to explore and respect the concerns of others. Remember that transitional thinking is characterised by the consideration of different possibilities. This, at the absolute minimum, is what you should be aiming for.

One of the ways to demonstrate your positive attitudes and values relating to care is to seize opportunities to discuss care philosophy with your supervisor and other senior staff. If you demonstrate an enquiring and respectful interest in what is being done, you are much more likely to convey favourable impressions to others. Students are usually well evaluated where both compassion and humility are combined. To evaluate others as 'wrong', 'stupid' or 'naive' is likely to convey an arrogant attitude.

Whatever you claim regarding your attitudes and values, though, remember that deeds speak louder than words. Have you worn your uniform correctly? Have you been punctual? Have you shown a due degree of flexibility as regards what others need to do? Are you polite? How do others know that you are listening attentively to what they tell you? The patterns of shifts that you complete as a student on placement are a foretaste of what work will feel like. For nurses to trust you as a colleague, they must feel sure that you will attend on time and work with interest on what the team is trying to achieve. Part of contextual thinking, which you learned about in Chapter 3, is associated with work and practice ethic, getting the job done in a professional, effective and efficient manner.

If you have received critical commentary as regards your attitudes or values, I recommend the following:

- Clarify what, specifically, the assessor is referring to, without challenging the assessment itself: 'Can you help me with that point? I need to understand which colleagues I have seemed dismissive of.'
- Ask how the assessment was made. It is unusual for an assessor to reach this judgement by themselves, so ask whether they have conferred with others before reaching the judgement. A professional assessor will usually have conferred on such matters, realising how unsettling such an evaluation can seem.
- Ask whether you demonstrated any positive behaviour, that which seemed to convey a better impression of your attitudes and values. It is quite reasonable to ask for assurance that the balance of your behaviour has been considered too.
- Take the criticism away and think about it before raising your concerns with your practice supervisor or link tutor. If you wish to raise points about these matters, write them down and acknowledge both strengths and weaknesses in your practice. Confronting assessors with the challenge 'You're all wrong!' is unconvincing and suggests a lack of insight.

Chapter summary

There are several key messages in this chapter. Learning in clinical practice is different to the explorative and risk-free enquiry of campus, sometimes intense, and you must be an active and organised learner. You help to shape the learning experience by working with your supervisor. But learning in this setting need not seem chaotic. If you approach the placement well organised and ready to study that which you observe, using questions such as those I suggest, there is every chance that you will extract important insights from your placement. Not only will you discover what counts as a problem, how solutions are negotiated, but you will learn a good deal about clinicians and their reasoning templates. You will learn a great deal about healthcare systems and how service is conceived.

In clinical practice, you learn about teamwork and professional etiquette. You are socialised to a healthcare system that strives to personalise care wherever possible but which also must make the most efficient use of finite resources. Clinicians work with imperfect knowledge (e.g. before diagnosis of an illness). They work accordingly with processes that are designed to make a problem known and to suggest solutions which assist anxious patients. Because you need to understand how the team proceeds, the practice supervisor is an important guide.

You need to carefully consider the feedback you receive. It can seem bruising to face criticism about something you thought you were good at; but remember that contexts change, and what worked in one place might not be appropriate in another. Nursing is a profession that works within contexts. The feedback will usually be carefully considered and supported afterwards with a review of what might improve matters.

Activities: brief outline answers

Activity 6.2 Critical thinking (page 101)

I would start by explaining that care seems to stretch in all directions at once – I need to chop it up in ways that seem open to analysis. After that, I hope to understand the circumstances in which the episode arose, its context. That might seem very familiar to clinical staff, but I still need to study it. Then I want to search for patterns of activity, what is happening. So, I ask whether what I saw or heard was accompanied by other things, those closely related that might help shape the episode. I am also interested in causes and consequences, cause and effect, how what you said or did with the patient seem to affect things. Lastly, I need to understand what that tells us about care, what helps the patient. Once I have understood that, I will perhaps be in a better position to write up a reflection.

Activity 6.3 Reflection (page 103)

I suspect that some of the cognitive dissonance problems that you will meet centre on providing enough individual care to patients when others require your time too. They will centre on time and energy: 'If only I could spend more time understanding the patient's needs and perspectives!' There are also likely to be compromises between protocol/policy and what you have read about in research findings: 'Why can't the clinical team just use the latest research?' Of course, research may not have been robust, scaled to practice, or related to a particular context. In these circumstances, it is tempting to side with campus and to judge practice as a place that struggles to catch up with best practice. You resolve the cognitive dissonance by siding with one perspective.

In reality, however, professionalism lies somewhere in the middle. Care is a contract and parties must have realistic expectations of the other; frequently, there are roles for both to play. Do not underestimate the importance of this search for equilibrium – sustaining a lifelong and satisfying career in nursing may depend upon it.

Further reading

Standing, M. (2020) *Clinical Judgement and Decision Making in Nursing*, 4th edition. London: SAGE/Learning Matters.

This valuable book leads the reader through different ways of thinking about clinical decision-making and explains how an understanding of ethics, reflection and priorities can lead to better decision-making. Of all the things that can seem mysterious and awe-inspiring in practice, it is the decision-making of experienced practitioners that is the most significant. Reading about these processes is therefore a valuable adjunct to clinical placement learning.

Useful websites

A visit to the ScienceDirect website (**www.sciencedirect.com**) affords you access to a number of free-to-access healthcare articles. Of particular interest, however, is the following:

Hashemiparast, M., Negarandeh, R. and Theofanidis, D. (2019) Exploring the barriers of utilizing theoretical knowledge in clinical settings: a qualitative study. *International Journal of Nursing Sciences*, 6(4): 399–405.

The authors catalogue a range of confidence issues relating to using theory in practice. Equally significant (I think) is the unwritten assumption that theory is fit for purpose. It is worth speculating on the relative roles of theory and practice. Does theory serve practice or does it direct practice? Is theory born out of practice need or from another place, perhaps professional philosophy?

Chapter 7 Making use of electronic media

Chapter aims

After reading this chapter, you will be able to:

- summarise the ways in which electronic media communication influences critical thinking;
- identify the ways in which electronic media might enhance the quality of your learning;
- explore personal interests regarding the use of electronic media in support of learning;
- identify ways in which tutors provide feedback on assignments and how this could be used;
- prepare appropriate contributions to electronic forums associated with your course of studies.

Introduction

There are excellent reasons for some of your studies to be completed using electronic media. Here are just a few:

- Recorded lectures and skill demonstrations can be run online, enabling you to pause and rerun video clips so that you can check over the points made. It is efficient for a university to use recorded lectures, freeing up more time for lecturers to run seminars or study groups with you and for staff to complete research.

- Interactive study online (e.g. wikis, electronic classrooms) acquaints you with technology. A significant amount of technology is now shaping healthcare (e.g. the use of Skype or Zoom for clinical consultation). Technology is transforming what it means to be a healthcare consumer (Marx and Padmanabhan, 2020).
- Electronic resources significantly increase your access to knowledge, both within the library and through websites, and beyond (Shakeel and Bhatti, 2018). However, you will need to be discriminating in what you read and what you deduce from different media.
- Electronic media offers the possibility of podcasts, short elements of audio teaching (Blum, 2018). While you may consume these, studying what a lecturer argues, you might also learn to make them yourself. A good deal of patient teaching, for example, could be designed in the form of podcasts (e.g. coping with diet and diabetes).
- An electronic facility such as Skype enables you to network with other nurses in your chosen field, including those working overseas. Networking increases your fund of valuable information (Dickson et al., 2016).
- Your study notes, portfolio, and course or placement reports can be stored electronically using a cloud facility. At its simplest, this means carrying around less bulky notebooks and folders.
- During a period of pandemic, or indeed other illness or personal incapacity, you can sustain portions of your study, keeping up to date with the lectures and discussions presented online.

Activity 7.1 Critical enquiry

Conduct a brief enquiry now to explore how technology aids skills instruction. Visit YouTube (**www.youtube.com**) and type in the search 'clinical skills demonstration'. You will discover a number of skill demonstrations on offer. Review two or three of the videos available and assess what this media adds to a clinical skills demonstration. Are there any cautionary points to note?

Some brief thoughts are given at the end of the chapter.

Electronic media is not a perfect platform for all learning. Nursing is a very interpersonal profession, and we need to engage with people face to face and in real time (Conroy, 2018). Electronic media struggles to simulate the conditions of healthcare practice. Face-to-face role play, for instance, is arguably better than electronic discussion. Interacting online with study group peers, either in a forum or using a wiki, is a different psychological experience. In a classroom, the words you share in a discussion are said and gone. In an interactive online discussion, they are often typed in or audio-recorded, which can leave you feeling a little more exposed to scrutiny by others: 'I wish I hadn't said that!'

Activity 7.2 Reflection

Pause now to reflect on how you view technology learning and healthcare. If we divide electronic resources into those that deliver information (e.g. library texts, recorded lectures) and those that require interaction on your part (e.g. an electronic forum), which seems the more exciting or useful, and which seems the more challenging?

My answers to this activity are given at the end of the chapter.

In this chapter, we examine what is involved in learning using different electronic media, and I make suggestions about how you can derive benefit from them. To illustrate critical thinking and reflection in action, I refer to two case studies. The first of these is the handling of emailed assignment feedback. The second relates to electronic forums and concerns the development of arguments around best nursing practice.

Email

Your use of electronic media (e.g. Facebook, Twitter) in the past may have been linked to things such as social networking and text messaging. Nurses vary widely in their electronic media experience, and some may feel less electronic media 'savvy' than others (Ahmad et al., 2018). Upon joining a nursing course, though, it is likely that you will be linked to a course web page within the university, and you will have an email account set up for you so that you can communicate with your tutor, the library and study group colleagues. Email extends the campus in significant ways. Through email, you may receive a 'study group message' from your tutor.

Just as there is etiquette associated with the use of electronic forums ('netiquette'), so there is one associated with the use of email for educational purposes. Beyond the usual caution that to type in CAPITALS is rude (it equates to shouting), there are other, equally important rules associated with what is and is not to be discussed using email. For example, you may discuss a draft piece of coursework with your tutor by email, but to do so with a study buddy is to risk censure. This is because of university rules concerning academic collusion and the need to ensure that work is not plagiarised.

Wikis

You may not have encountered a wiki before, but it can be described simply as an electronic space where individuals make contributions that add to the understanding of a subject (Trocky and Buckley, 2016). Individuals type their entry to the wiki in a text box, check what they have written, and then post it to the wiki space on the course web page. The purpose of a wiki is to add layers of information – extra interpretations of what has been posted as the subject of the wiki. So, for example, a tutor might ask you to build a collective explanation of 'rehabilitation'. In this way, as each student adds a small contribution, an extended definition of the concept emerges. The wiki remains online as a reference resource for students to draw on later.

Wikis are used in different ways. Sometimes they form the basis of an electronic seminar where you discuss what has been revealed by the information collated. At other times, though, the wiki simply acts as a resource that you have built jointly on an important concept. It is something that you can return to in later modules. Rehabilitation, for example, is a recurring theme relevant in many fields of healthcare work, cancer care, mental illness and trauma care.

Activity 7.3   Critical thinking

Imagine now a concept that you think might be explored using a wiki. It should be one that is open to the experience of others, their knowledge of people and practice, as well as literature or research. Why might it be exciting to explore concepts in this way?

An outline answer is given at the end of this chapter.

Electronic forums

Most courses offer electronic forums, which are places where students and tutors can communicate with one another, either asynchronously (i.e. over time) or synchronously (i.e. at a designated time) (Adams et al., 2015). Quite often an electronic forum is used to conduct a seminar where you mutually review the articles that you have read. As with wikis, you access the relevant electronic forum using your membership or student identification number and individual password, a process that ensures the relative privacy of discussions within that space. Individual forum discussions are connected to course modules, and postings made there may demonstrate your 'attendance' or even contribute to course marks achieved.

In the forum, a series of individual discussions is initiated (often by the tutor); as each student adds responses of their own, a 'thread' develops. At different points, the tutor may tidy up the thread, editing material so as to ensure the final record of discussion remains comprehensible to all. Electronic forums are, of course, rather different from the tutorials you might share in a classroom. For one thing, a record exists of what each student has contributed. This can seem a little worrying if you equate conversations here with records of performance. It takes a little while to appreciate that most forums are places of honest and thoughtful speculation.

Electronic classrooms

Electronic forums are valuable, especially the asynchronous ones, as you have the opportunity to visit them when it suits you best. Nonetheless, the conversations can seem a little slow or stilted. For this reason, many universities use electronic classrooms. Electronic classrooms are designed to function as tutorials within the online environment, and they offer significant benefits when it comes to managing study time (Andrew et al., 2015). There are no car parking or public transport expenses associated with attending these tutorials, but you will need access to a modern computer that runs the latest software, as well as a headset microphone, so that you can participate successfully.

You join the electronic classroom using a preset web address (a URL) and log in with your membership or student identification number and individual password. What then appears is a whiteboard screen upon which you or your tutor will be able to draw diagrams, make lists and sketch flow charts. Beside the whiteboard screen, there is a series of control features with which you need to acquaint yourself using university training sessions. Commonly, these features include:

- a facility to ask questions or make points (using your microphone);
- the opportunity to vote in debates or in response to tutor questions;
- a facility to view streamed audio/video material;
- the opportunity to visit other web addresses using hyperlinks provided (highlighted words that take you to a new place if you click on these with your mouse);
- a facility to move to a 'breakout' room where you conduct small group discussions.

Electronic classrooms usually require a little technical preparation (configuring your computer) and some discipline (especially in the use of microphones). They can seem unfamiliar, insofar as you do not necessarily see the faces of other students. Against that, however, they provide real-time interactive learning for students who might not be studying on campus. Using an electronic classroom, you develop computer-facilitated conferencing skills that may be important in your future health-care work.

Case study: Making good use of feedback

We come now to the first of four case studies within this chapter. As part of your coursework, it is possible that you will submit both formative assignments (those not awarded a grade) and summative assignments (those that are grade-bearing) electronically to your tutor, as well as receiving your feedback in a similarly paperless way. Electronic submission has the advantage that you can obtain a record of the assignment being submitted on time. One of the other key advantages of an electronically submitted assignment is that the tutor can give you both summary feedback (as an end of work commentary) and feedback in the form of textual annotations which you can read as part of an attachment emailed back to you (see Figure 7.1).

Children have particular difficulties expressing pain. Younger ones have a more limited vocabulary to describe the pain and may use general terms like 'tummy' to refer to its location. They don't have a clear sense of time and may struggle to describe the duration of the pain. MacGrath (1989) [McGrath (1990) in your reference list[ER1]] explains that nurses have to use parents to help interpret the pain. Parents are familiar with the way in which a child expresses themselves and can help determine whether pain may be a problem, for example when the child seems distracted and unable to concentrate on what they are doing[ER2]. Children have just as much pain as the rest of us and it's wrong to assume that they don't feel pain in the same way as adults[You need a reference here and perhaps to consider making this a separate paragraph. This paragraph is all about the expression of pain and your last point is about the incidence or nature of pain encountered].

Comment [ER1]: Are there more recent references that you could use?

Comment [ER2]: Do you think there are any circumstances when we need to be more cautious about relying upon a parent to help interpret a child's pain? If you are unsure, why not look up 'Munchausen by proxy' syndrome?

Figure 7.1 Examples of track change and margin note commentary feedback

Figure 7.1 illustrates two forms of feedback on a single paragraph extract from a student's assignment answer. The first is called 'track changes' and is presented here as underlined text that appears within the body of the essay work. In the first instance, track changes have been used to correct the presentation of a reference. The adjustment shows the correct spelling of the author name and queries the date of publication. In the second track change, the tutor provides guidance on both the

(Continued)

(Continued)

referencing of the work and the planning of coherent paragraphs. The second form of feedback consists of marginal annotations using the 'comment' feature. ER in this instance stands for 'educational reviewer', although initials can be changed to reflect the name of the tutor. It does not stand for 'error', because some margin annotations might be used to congratulate you on your work.

While the volume and complexity of written feedback on an assignment answer may vary, good feedback remains unambiguous. There are no unexplained '?s' and '!s' dotted around that leave you to guess what the tutor means. Some questions then follow: What purpose is the feedback fulfilling? How will you make sense of it? What will you do next?

The purpose of feedback

One purpose of feedback is to correct a misapprehension, whether it concerns a reference, a drug calculation or an assertion about ethical care (McCarthy et al., 2018). Corrections are often handled using track changes, with the tutor either deleting something and inserting the correct material or commenting on the deficits. But other feedback may have a more subtle function. Comment ER1 in Figure 7.1 is designed to prompt some further thought and enquiry. Sometimes feedback is more rhetorical and designed to illustrate the way in which the tutor is 'thinking aloud' (ER2). Tutors do not invariably expect you to respond to such remarks, but may leave them for further consideration. On occasions, the marginal commentary is intentionally provocative as well as rhetorical, as in this example: 'Perhaps we are naive to imagine what can be easily assessed. It is bound up with private experiences, memories and fears. I wonder what you think?'

Making sense of feedback

We need, then, to make sense of the tutor's feedback. Does it require a response on my part? Does it prompt some new work for me? However important a coursework mark or grade might seem, the commentary that accompanies your assignment answer is important too. Even if you have achieved a good mark, there is always something more to glean from the commentary provided. Why is this a good essay? Seeing the pass mark and heaving a sigh of relief are not enough. You need to ascertain what the tutor thinks you have learned here and what could remain to be achieved. For instance, does the tutor comment on the structure of your essay answer? Does the feedback highlight your ability to argue a case?

Doing something with feedback

While logistically tutors supporting large student groups cannot enter into protracted dialogue with every student, there is a strong case for corresponding further with your tutor in the following circumstances:

- where you have secured a poor grade and/or where the commentary suggests that you have misunderstood the question;
- where the commentary suggests a significant gap in your subject knowledge (that gap may prove important in later assessments);
- where the feedback has posed new questions to you (you wish to ask the tutor to help clarify a matter);
- where the tutor has suggested other possible lines of enquiry.

It is understandable to worry that you may inconvenience a busy tutor; but if they signal the above things, they really do welcome your follow-up enquiry. The conversations that follow on from the assignment feedback will help you to develop your powers of discrimination and argument formation.

Activity 7.4   Reflection

Reflect now on any assignment feedback that you have received to date and answer the following question:

- Did I use this to help develop my critical thinking or reflective practice?

If the answer is no, decide next why that was:

- Did the electronic form of communication put you off, making it seem impersonal?
- Or, on the contrary, did it make receiving feedback easier?

As this answer is based on your own reflection, there is no outline answer at the end of the chapter.

Case study: Making arguments in the forum

My second case example of electronic media-mediated learning concerns the use of electronic forums. Tutors use these forums for various purposes, including the development of study group conversations that track changes in your collective thinking (tutors

(Continued)

(Continued)

can archive forum discussions and later invite your group to revisit past reasoning).
Making contributions to the electronic forum can seem more difficult, though. I asked
Fatima to reflect on contributing to forums. She said:

> *I have enjoyed the different forums that we shared so far. To read other people's ideas
> is encouraging. But posting my ideas was more difficult. It was easy to support
> someone else, to say, 'Yes, I agree', but more difficult to suggest something of my own.
> I found myself thinking, 'This is not polite, to insist in this way to my colleagues.'*

Fatima's reflections are familiar to tutors. However, making arguments is necessary if
you are to advance your thinking. There is a need to formulate arguments and to test
them with supportive peers and an empathetic tutor. Happily, the system for posting
forum messages involves composition and there is a chance to review your posting
before you press 'send'. While most students do this to check their grammar and syntax, the greatest benefit of the pre-submission check is being able to consider whether
your points seem coherent and clear. No one in the forum expects perfection, especially in a synchronous discussion. No one anticipates that their comments will always
be supported either. Just as in other conversations, there will be some good points
made and some that seem more questionable. Making a clear argument, though, is
something that we can practise when we edit messages before they are posted.

Activity 7.5   Critical thinking

Imagine that you are engaged in a forum discussion about the right (or
otherwise) of individuals to end their own lives. The last posting made
by another student (John) expresses a deeply held religious conviction
that patients should not exercise such a right, and that to do so relieves
healthcare practitioners of the responsibility to deliver better end of life care.
Now it is your turn to offer something. Consider the three observations below
and decide which, if any, you might post to the forum. I discuss the merits of
each below but encourage you to evaluate them first:

1. I can see John's point regarding who should have the right to curtail a life,
    but it is fair to observe that significant numbers of people do not express
    a religious conviction and question whether there is an absolute law here.
    Patients are consumers. If we require patients to make choices in other
    areas, why are they not capable of making decisions about death?

2. One of the things that we wrestle with is how patients' decisions make
    us feel. Their actions seem to reflect on us: 'I ended my life because you
    couldn't help me.' This seems a terrible thing, and yet these are views
    that we can imagine patients holding.

3. The media debate concerning this topic is often about the intentions of those who facilitate death. If there are inheritance benefits being sought, or if the death of the person simply makes life more convenient for others, ending a life undermines dignity in society. But if the decision is truthfully about the relief of suffering, as well as acknowledging that quality of life has gone, perhaps we have to support carers.

As this answer is based on your own observation, there is no outline answer at the end of the chapter.

In Chapter 1, you were briefly introduced to the business of making arguments. Whether or not the above observations represent arguments is debatable, as we shall shortly discuss. But let me start first by indicating that seminar discussions and real-time electronic forums are often difficult places to make formal (philosophically logical, inductive) arguments. We are after all thinking on our feet. Arguments (those that we might agree upon) might emerge after some considerable discussion. One of the reasons that Fatima might find it uncomfortable offering responses in an electronic forum could be that she senses her offerings are 'just opinions'. I would suggest that it is premature in such discussions to imagine that you must all venture logical arguments. Oftentimes we creep up on better explanations of what is happening through discussion. One of the functions of a forum, as well as the guidance of tutors, is to help you learn to argue.

So, let us look at each of the observations in turn. Arguments comprise a case (that which you advocate) and the premises which you believe support it. Not only must each premise be factually correct, but they must fit in a clear way with the case (Pape, 2019). Better arguments usually include the word 'because'. For example, patients struggle to secure a right to end their lives (the case) because: (a) regulatory authorities fear that pressure may be placed upon individuals to curtail their lives; (b) religious groups argue that such a route represents a sin; and (c) those close to the dying person might act not in the interest of the patient. Here, (a), (b) and (c) are the premises. In an argument, premises should be open to scrutiny and their fit with the case open to debate. You could, for example, look at religious teaching on suicide.

Observation 1 is, I suggest, a speculative opinion. The case is that patients have a right to make choices about their death. For this observation to start working as an argument, we would need premises about patients' decision-making rights. Nonetheless, it is a valuable starting observation. A tutor might say, 'What evidence is there that we allow patients to make big decisions about their health?' You see, it is about logic. It might be illogical to deny patients a choice to end their lives if we give them responsibility for most other things about their lives (informed consent).

What about observation 2? This is an observation about cost, is it not? Specifically, it is a fear that if patients were to elect for voluntary euthanasia, we would have to confront that it felt like an indictment of our efforts to care. Strictly speaking, there is not a case – it too is speculative. This is another facet of dying and euthanasia, but it is an observation about the emotional cost to us of the patient's decision. There might be an argument here if you ventured something about why clinicians are circumspect about promoting euthanasia as a right.

Observation 3 seems a speculation with an argument struggling to get out. The case is (roughly) that the debate on euthanasia rests upon the inferred motives of those who are complicit in the patient's decision to end their life. If the motive is noble (to end suffering and despair), then euthanasia might be contemplated. But if the motive is, say, pecuniary (a relative inherits the patient's home), then that undermines the case that euthanasia is in the patient's own interests. An interesting debate could emerge from this regarding how we might exclude the selfish motives of those who facilitate euthanasia.

What can we say, then, about the business of contributing within electronic forums? First, it seems necessary to accept that forums are not the same as face-to-face seminars. They leave a record, and it is for this reason that you will naturally wish to compose your contributions carefully. Second, successful forums are permissive and allow that arguments might develop within and through them. You will make several observations and the clarity of matters will improve as the group takes stock of what has been posted. It is OK to 'feel your way' in these matters. Your tutor has a key role here, helping to sum up points. Third, discussions held in electronic forums are not and should not be reputation busters. Your tutor should make this clear at the outset; otherwise, trust will not grow within the study group.

Case study: Interacting successfully within the electronic classroom

In the third case study, we turn to successful learning within the electronic classroom environment. Although you have already learned valuable principles while reading about learning from lectures and seminars, there are some subtle variations here that you need to be aware of. Much of what you need to consider now relates to attending sensitively to the needs of fellow learners, as well as making the technology work for everyone. As you cannot necessarily see other class participants, you have to imagine how they feel as they interface with the classroom using a computer.

Let us start with strategy. Your strategy should begin before the class itself and should ensure that you are well prepared to play an inquisitive role during the session. Preparation begins by noting on what date and at what time the class session begins. It can be very disruptive to join the class late and then try to catch up on what has already been done. To ensure that you can contribute fully, it is necessary to do a brief computer check. Most of the electronic classroom platforms have a log-on wizard facility, which allows you to check that you can hear the audio output clearly and test that your microphone is working well. Running these sound checks well in advance should ensure that there is much less chance you will inconvenience others. Familiarise yourself with the various control functions at your command within the electronic classroom. Check to see that you can turn your microphone on and off (the screen icon will change). You need to have your microphone off when you are not speaking, otherwise your open-channel microphone might block a fellow student.

The classroom is likely to have a separate response box where you can type in text (e.g a question). Conduct a trial run before the class to ensure that your typed text appears in the box as expected. Your tutor will be able to see this while running the session. Do not assume, however, that all such typed text responses are instantly acted on. Responses to such student queries may be saved for a summing-up point. Identify whether you are able to indicate your understanding of the session using emoticons (smiling or frowning faces). Your tutor might rely on these to determine the pace and direction that the class takes.

Attending to the class itself requires a little extra thought as well. Remember that you will be seated before a computer screen, possibly many miles from the university itself. The tutor cannot readily see if you are listening intently or whether you look interested or bored. So, I recommend that you:

- have a notebook and pencil to hand (you may wish to compose queries or reflections carefully before posting these within the electronic classroom);
- have refreshments to hand (avoid spilling liquids on the computer, however);
- use the 'out of the room' icon to indicate when you are not present in class.

Class sizes vary, but a key consideration is to post responses, either typed or audio, that seem constructive and do not dominate the discussion. Remember that you cannot see the scowls of other students in this environment. So, monitor whether others have already typed in questions or reflections within the text box, and where possible save your points for the frequent 'Are you all happy?' breaks that experienced tutors tend to use. If you wish to refer to something specifically, note down the location in your notebook: 'I have a query about slide 4 in the PowerPoint presentation ...'

Where students agree, classroom sessions are archived (i.e. they are recorded) so that you and your fellow students can access them again later. If this has not been agreed, however, you will need to make notes as you proceed through the class. PowerPoint presentations are often sent to you by the tutor for later reference. Anticipate, however, that at the end of the session, you may be asked to conclude what you understood. Having notes to hand will help you to do that and to indicate what you hope to follow up study on. As with face-to-face lectures, the notes made here are likely to be brief and will need expansion after the class has finished.

Case study: Evaluating website information

The final case study within this chapter concerns the critical evaluation of website information. Quite commonly within electronic learning, you will be invited to conduct a search on the internet and will then be asked to critically examine what you found there. Chapter 8 provides additional guidance on the critical examination of evidence, but I also need to add some remarks on the internet as a source of knowledge. The internet represents a new frontier of information, much of it unregulated and some of it arguably spurious (Jordan and Chambers, 2017). While the internet can be liberating, it can also be misguiding.

The internet is comprised of service providers that offer search facilities to different website addresses (URLs). Each website offers a range of content and authors. In many instances, the website providers will be the content authors as well. So, for example, if you go to the website for the NMC (**www.nmc-uk.org**), the content provided will be authored by the NMC itself, or its approved researchers or consultants. In other instances, however, a website may provide the facility for different authors to post their content. The website owners note that the content found there does not necessarily reflect their views. One of the strengths of the internet is that it provides a forum for a wide range of views and insights, some of them cutting-edge. There is a minimum of regulation, save for that demanded by governments to protect the vulnerable and limit criminal activity.

The first questions that you should pose when you find internet information, then, are: Who are the authors? Who makes the claims presented here? In many instances, there are no authors named in website information; the conventions of published books or articles do not apply. It is then necessary to examine what they argue (searching for possible bias) and to determine whether the author's perspectives may have been shaped by the owner of the website. For example, you find a paper on the part played by sugar in the human diet that makes a number of assertions about why it is beneficial. Counterarguments about the risks of excess sugar consumption are not aired. The paper is found on the website of an organisation with close associations with several processed food manufacturers. Caution may then be required, and you might question whether the information found is impartial.

A further important question to ask regarding internet information is: When was it published? When you reference a website in your work, you detail the date that the site was accessed. What is also important, though, is to determine how old the information found there is. When was it published on the site, or indeed previously elsewhere? The best papers included within websites have both author details and details about when the paper was uploaded to the website. Many others, however, will lack one or more of these details, and then you will need to be circumspect about whether you can recommend this resource within your review. If the information was integral to the website itself (rather than an embedded paper), you might check the last date that the website was updated. This is sometimes stated within the 'home' page.

Activity 7.6   Research and evidence-based practice

Choose a subject to research on the internet – so much the better if this relates to a controversial subject, such as the causes of obesity, the rights of a particular patient group, cigarette smoking, or similar.

Use the facilities of your internet service provider to identify relevant websites and choose one of these to scrutinise in greater depth. How easy was it to ascertain who authored the website information and any affiliations that they had? Check whether the information provided seems to support the stated position or mission of the website owners (often expressed as 'our mission' or 'about us'). Check to see whether the website provides information about when the site was last updated and against what, if any, criteria.

As this answer is based on your own observation, there is no outline answer at the end of the chapter.

In examining websites as possible sources of information, the appropriate attitude is one of healthy scepticism (Jordan and Chambers, 2017). It is not necessarily the case that the information found is not valuable, but without details of its origin it is harder to check for bias. In healthcare, as elsewhere, commercial, ideological and political influences may play a role in shaping what is provided. As a critical consumer of this information, you will need to ask questions about what interest the information might serve – whether it was provided for your needs or those of others.

Chapter summary

In this chapter, I began with the argument that electronic media has much to offer learning, but some careful thought is required when using it. The way you reason using electronic media will be different from reasoning in class. This is not to suggest, however, that these media in some way undermine the critical thinking and reflection that can operate here. The quality of feedback possible with an electronically submitted assignment, the excitement that can be generated in an electronic classroom, the richness of information on the internet, and the depth of debate possible within an electronic forum can be exceptional. The very fact that you can access conversations at times to suit you, and that there is space to compose your answers with care that is not available in a real-time face-to-face conversation, highlights the critical thinking opportunities here.

(Continued)

(Continued)

Electronic media is not without challenges, though, and you may have observed within this chapter just how different this communication can seem. For some, it feels artificial, especially if students are private and contemplative in nature. If electronic learning environments are used without clear thought, the reputation of electronic learning quickly deteriorates. It is at its best where the tutor marshals fascinating resources to which the class has prompt access, which then form the focus of attention for discussion. Tutors are becoming adept in creating welcoming and supportive electronic learning environments. They recognise the anxieties that can lurk as you prepare your first postings, and they know that to contribute to something which remains 'on record' undermines the confidence of some. Acknowledging these concerns, they arrange feedback and summarise discussions in ways that demonstrate tolerance, an appreciation of your efforts, and a commitment to imaginative new ways to learn.

Activities: brief outline answers

Activity 7.1 Critical enquiry (page 109)

Well-filmed and adequately narrated skill demonstrations can be a boon in nurse education, but there are caveats to note. The first is that skills and procedures operate in the context of clinical policies and with resources that might be different in your healthcare system, so it is important to check how well the demonstration works with local requirements. Many principles expressed within demonstrations (e.g. cross-infection control) are universal, but it is still worth checking the published date that the item was added to the internet to ensure that what you study is reasonably current. Check whether the demonstration includes any close-up camerawork, which might be important when demonstrating skills such as wound suturing, for instance. Does the demonstrator offer a rationale for the sequence of work done, and is there adequate recognition of the patient's needs?

Activity 7.2 Reflection (page 110)

While finding your way around the electronic facilities offered by a large university library can be daunting for some (delivered information), in my experience it is the interactive electronic learning activities that worry students the most. This is because a complex media has been inserted between those communicating. We are less able to monitor the reactions of others to what we contribute. All mediated forms of communication take time to adjust to. For example, it probably took you a little while to get used to texting abbreviations on a mobile phone when you first started. Much of nursing is interpersonal, and there are good reasons to replicate that in nurse education. Technology should not become a media that dominates learning to the detriment of demonstrating that which we must master in practice. Nonetheless, it would be unwise to dismiss the many merits of electronic learning media. It is capable of bringing vast amounts of knowledge to you and speeding up your enquiry.

Activity 7.3 Critical thinking (page 111)

My example of a wiki topic is entirely topical in 2021 as the world wrestles with the Covid-19 pandemic. It concerns what is understood about the virus, its spread, and the risks for human beings. This is a topic that is almost daily streaming new information, especially about risks to different groups of patients. You may have personal experience of the virus and revised your notion of risk because of it. It is exactly the sort of topic that lends itself to wiki development.

Further reading

Flyverbom, M. (2019) *The Digital Prism: Transparency and Managed Visibilities in a Datafied World.* Cambridge: Cambridge University Press.

Mikkel Flyverbom reminds us that digital technology is increasingly intruding into every aspect of modern life, sometimes obtrusively so. The argument runs that the digital revolution increases connectivity between people but diminishes privacy. It is well worth thinking about, for instance, with regard to patient records and the safety and reputation of healthcare professionals. Is there a case to limit such technology, and if so when is that point reached?

Littlejohn, A. and Hood, N. (2018) *Reconceptualizing Learning in the Digital Age: The (Un)democratising Potential of MOOCs.* New York: Springer.

Once upon a time, distance and open learning universities were distinct from those that taught on campus. However, the differences between the two now blur – your electronic-based learning could happen in either institution. What blurs matters further are massive open online courses (MOOCs), which are presented by universities and studied by a much wider variety of students. Pause to consider, though, what happens when learners in your group come from a much wider background and study your module to different ends. The design of education is a principal interest for your tutor, but you too are in the midst of a technological revolution and that affects how you are invited to think.

Useful websites

I want to suggest two useful resources found on YouTube (**www.youtube.com**). The first is for any of you who feel lost by the multitude of information available on the internet, entitled *How I Learn Things Online (Way More Efficiently)* by Nathaniel Drew (**www.youtube.com/watch?v=rVmMbMa3ncI**). Nathaniel is a photographer and an enthusiastic speaker on the personal organisation of enquiry. You will have access to dedicated university library resources, but it is still valuable to contemplate what the internet offers. If you venture there, then your enquiries will need to be disciplined. Nathaniel researches photography, but his enquiry principles still hold good for healthcare.

The second resource is entitled *How to Use Zoom for Remote and Online Learning* by Flipped Classroom Tutorials (**www.youtube.com/watch?v=9guqRELB4dg**). Universities use a variety of platforms to deliver online classroom teaching, and this is just one of them. What it does do, however, is to help you understand how the tutor manages such an environment. There is no reason why a group of nurses cannot band together to use such a platform for professional update purposes. Sue (our case study registered nurse) helps to run a journal club using this technology. Each takes a turn running the monthly meetings and every session reviews at least one research article.

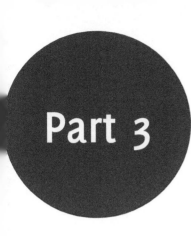

Part 3

Expressing critical thought and reflection

Chapter 8   Critiquing evidence-based literature

Chapter aims

After reading this chapter, you will be able to:

- outline the different ways in which evidence might be defined;
- referring to paradigms, summarise why evidence needs to be critically analysed in different ways;
- discuss validity, reliability, transferability and authenticity as key criteria by which to examine evidence;
- use insights from the ongoing debates about better research evidence to explain why the application of knowledge to practice is not always easy.

Introduction

In a healthcare world where there is an increasing amount of information, theory and evidence, two overarching questions should exercise our thinking. The first is: To what extent are theory and evidence applicable in practice? This is an important question to consider because not all information is realistically utilisable in healthcare. Some philosophical material, for example, is designed to help conceptualise what nursing might be like (Nelson-Brantley et al., 2019). Person-centred care writers make recommendations for practice but might concede that only a percentage of the ideal practice is possible now. For person-centred care to work entirely, not only must healthcare be amply resourced, but it would have to operate with patients eager to partner nurses in care (Price, 2019b). If we do not ask questions about the utility of information for practice, we risk cognitive dissonance.

The second and more discrete question concerns the nature of evidence and how we can best evaluate it. We think of evidence as a superior kind of information, although it too has limits (Murphy, 2019). If evidence were all of one kind, then our evaluative work would be much easier. We would simply work with a series of universal questions to check whether the evidence is sound. In this chapter, though, you will discover that evidence is not all of one kind and that there are then different questions to be asked about each of these.

The importance of utility

Periodically within this book, I have encouraged you to ask whether ideas are realisable in practice. This is not to simply promote cynicism; it is instead to acknowledge limits to the uses that particular information can reasonably be put. Let me illustrate. In the 1990s, I developed a theory of body image to help nurses understand how patients dealing with a wide variety of injuries and illnesses might experience their bodies in new ways (Price, 1990). The implication was that if we could understand patient distress, then we could develop supportive measures to help them cope.

The simple triangular model describing how body image is experienced proved very successful. It was a useful heuristic (explanatory) device. But the theory of altered body image care (what came next) proved harder to action. This was because it assumed some counselling ability of the nurse, adequate time to explore the experience, and recognition that body image care had to be shared across different agencies. Nurses in hospitals had to refer patients on to others in the community. An acutely distressed patient might have to be referred to a psychologist. The key point was that the theory had value but also limits. Body image care was often therapy, and debates then arose about how to ensure its continuity.

I share this illustration to emphasise that information shared in many areas of nursing is a work in progress. Something that started as a means of explaining a phenomenon (altered body image) began to expand into a guide on how to practise to therapeutic effect. The problem was that the theory had finite utility. However compelling it was philosophically and professionally, it was limited by issues associated with healthcare resources and by practitioner skills.

As you discuss theory and research evidence on campus, there is a short series of questions that you can use to check the practice utility of what is promoted. In the event that you conclude the information has finite practice utility, it may still have purpose elsewhere. For example, the information may inform the professional philosophy of nursing. It might be used by nurse leaders to argue for a different allocation of healthcare resources. Just because information is difficult to utilise now does not mean that it does not have professional merit. Nursing is dynamic.

Here are the suggested questions:

- *What assumptions are made about patients and their next of kin?* Care is fundamentally a collaborative activity. We proceed with the patient's insight and informed consent, so this becomes an acid test of what theory or evidence can be used with confidence in practice.
- *What assumptions are made about the role of the nurse and their skills?* Some of the theory and evidence that you meet on campus might easily be within the remit and the skill set of an advanced practitioner or consultant nurse. Other information might be usable by a range of nurses.
- *What assumptions are made about the range and appropriate focus of a healthcare service?* This is quite tricky as in some regards service provision might be confused. Different agencies might do different things, and different hospitals, for example, might work with different protocols. Nevertheless, the question is an important one. What service emphasis should be placed on public health, reducing the risk of illness versus treating people who have already fallen ill?
- *What assumptions are made about interprofessional working?* The remit of nursing has expanded in recent decades, but there remains role overlap and gaps that can make care decision-making, consultation and collaboration more difficult (Goldsberry, 2018).

Activity 8.1 Reflection

Pause now to reflect on any recent clinical placements that you have completed. Would the above questions help you to clarify why there may have seemed to be gaps between theory and practice? What if practice dominated the nursing syllabus entirely? What if theory was the only driver of that which is taught?

A brief reflection on the last questions is given at the end of this chapter.

The nature of evidence

We can turn now to the second question and the nature of evidence. To explore this subject, I return to the four case study nursing students who we first met in Chapter 1. Each has searched for and engaged with evidence within the healthcare literature. But as we shall see below, critical thinking – when it is applied to evidence – is not straight-forward. Evidence is neither a neutral nor a straightforward concept, and the way in which evidence is defined may influence how it is then evaluated.

Activity 8.2   Critical thinking

Below I set out the opening definitions of evidence that Stewart, Fatima, Raymet and Gina have used to search for information. I asked them to illustrate their points, referring to the topic of pain and its management. As you can see, they are quite different, and as a result different sorts of literature might be found.

Decide which of the following definitions of evidence seem most convincing to you.

As this answer is based on your own observation, there is no outline answer at the end of the chapter.

Case study: Four definitions of 'evidence'

Gina: I've always thought of evidence as that which science, and in particular experimental research or randomised controlled trials, produces. What dis-tinguishes evidence from mere information is that the knowledge has been secured by design; there is a rigorous method to the work, and we can evalu-ate that. So, for me, there is an emphasis on pain interventions, medication and other treatments that might make a discernible difference.

Fatima: Maybe! But you're missing something here – evidence isn't restricted to research. Audits, patient satisfaction surveys, case studies of unusual patient situations and needs, what we did to look after them, that counts as evidence too! Pain is individual, so we need a wide-ranging appreciation of it.

Raymet: So what about the evidence of your own eyes, then? If reflection doesn't produce a sort of evidence too, aren't we missing out on something? Not everything can be examined in a piece of research. Nurses accumulate insights into pain, the emotional as well as the physical sort, and that needs to be considered too.

Stewart: Perhaps, then, evidence is that which you can measure, that which you can quantify. Other sorts of information are still important, but we shouldn't try to make evidence stretch so far, to serve every situation. We need evidence and patient stories – their narratives about coping with pain. Evidence, though, that should be apolitical, shouldn't it? It should be produced by those who don't have a particular axe to grind about healthcare and how care should be!

It might not surprise you to learn that evidence has been defined in all of the above ways, from either something quite distinct from other classes of knowledge to something that embraces a wide range of experience and insight (Ellis, 2019). Here, I suggest that evidence might be considered to be information that for the individual, group or organisation has greater authority than some other forms of knowledge, but which still requires scrutiny before it can be appropriately used.

Debates about what represents best evidence are not always solely about judging how the evidence has been secured. They are sometimes about what knowledge nurses should use, as well as what should be the proper study and the basis of nursing practice. If we research human experiences (e.g. that of the patient), then we may produce evidence that can tell us things about how nursing might be experienced, but we might not be able to predict outcomes for large groups of patients.

When the world-famous Cochrane Library was set up (**www.cochranelibrary.com**), it focused firmly upon a quite discrete form of evidence, concerned with interventions and cause-and-effect relationships. It focused upon treatments and what might be proven to work. Subsequently, the Cochrane Library has considered a rather more wide-ranging collection of evidence, which relates to experiences in healthcare as well. It has been accepted that evidence in healthcare needs to relate to different things, not only interventions, but analysis of experiences, problems, perceptions and preferences as well. The need to diversify the understanding of 'evidence' has grown as nurses and others have become increasingly concerned with healthcare quality, and quality has been understood in experiential as well as effectiveness terms (Holloway and Galvin, 2016).

I argue that evidence can only be critically evaluated when: (a) the original premises of the research or other knowledge are understood; and (b) we understand the conventions for critiquing that particular sort of evidence. You need to consider what your own attitude towards knowledge is, what is considered least and most important, and what you support as an essential resource upon which to draw when advancing nursing care (see Figure 8.1).

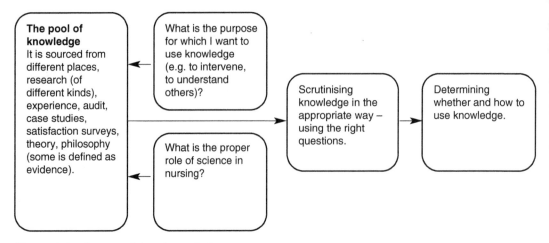

Figure 8.1   Approaching knowledge

Knowledge and how to know it

In 2012, Thomas Kuhn's classic 1962 book *The Structure of Scientific Revolutions*, one of the most influential philosophy texts of the last century, was reissued. Kuhn was eager to explain that there could be quite sudden and sometimes violent shifts in thinking, as well as what was accepted as truth. What represented incontrovertible evidence was, as it were, 'up for grabs'. One established way of understanding the world and conducting science therein (we call it a paradigm) could be disputed and replaced by another. The **positivist** paradigm centres upon the empirical world, that which can be manipulated and tested, and can be controlled – or at least managed – within laboratory and (to a lesser degree) clinical settings. The positivist paradigm draws heavily upon research methods associated with the natural sciences, and work concentrates on trying to demonstrate and measure cause-and-effect relationships, the limiting of researcher bias, and the testing of hypotheses (prediction of what would or would not be the case). Positivist science is classically associated with three things: accurate mapping, precise measurement and strategic manipulation (Creswell and Creswell, 2018). Well-designed positivist surveys map phenomena (e.g. anxiety traits) while experimental designs and randomised controlled trials manipulate things (e.g. the dosage of a particular drug given to patients).

Activity 8.3   Reflection

Pause at this stage to reflect upon the implications of the positivist conception of research for nursing. If scientific knowledge comprises what can be manipulated under controlled conditions, how well does this relate to nursing practice?

As this answer is based on your own observation, there is no outline answer at the end of the chapter.

The problem for many nurses was that the positivist paradigm, as well as its conception of knowledge, paid little attention to the practical conditions under which many people lived. The need to design studies that controlled for all undue influences (variables) meant that experiments could be exacting but they might not relate well to practical care situations. Within the healthcare world, there was little chance of controlling all the factors that could influence how individuals behaved, and in any case it was argued that people did not behave according to trait, but – in many instances – according to circumstance. Predicting human behaviour was problematic. As a result of this, a new paradigm or collective world view began to develop and compete with the positivist paradigm. This new world view is sometimes referred to as the **naturalistic** paradigm because researchers worked in social world conditions with fewer checks and controls on enquiry. The new paradigm is also sometimes referred to as the **interpretive** paradigm because there was a greater freedom for the researcher to interpret data, especially the experiences of others. But whatever we choose to call this new paradigm, it certainly includes a much-increased concern with insights into human experience (Zahavi and Martiny, 2019). The work of the researcher is much less about designing tests and more about enquiring within the social world in an authentic and sensitive fashion (e.g. interviews, observations in practice, case studies).

Activity 8.4   Critical thinking

What do you think the implications are of naturalistic paradigm reasoning for nursing and nursing research? For example, researchers working in this paradigm are very concerned to reveal the different ways in which patients experience the support of the nurse. But because the researcher is less concerned with controlling the data, the evidence resulting from this sort of research is often illustrative – it suggests what could be the case and expects the reader to determine whether their own experience matches what was reported.

As this answer is based on your own observation, there is no outline answer at the end of the chapter.

Debates continue between those who support positivism and those who support naturalism in nursing research (Garrett, 2016). Arguments are made about what does or does not constitute 'proper science'. The matter is still more complicated, however, by the emergence of a third competing paradigm that also produces research, the **critical theory** paradigm, which was founded upon the premise that knowledge is rarely neutral (Ryan, 2018). Knowledge inherently carries power and there are many people within the world who are eager to use it. Marxist researchers (who challenge class or other political elites) and feminist researchers (who argue that women and other disadvantaged groups are poorly served in society) work within this paradigm. These researchers propose that investigators use research to expose injustices and to empower others to take greater charge of their lives (Freeborn and Knafl, 2014). As a result, a lot of research in this paradigm has been described as action research, consisting of cycles of collaborative activity to improve the lot of disadvantaged groups in healthcare (Ryan, 2018).

Activity 8.5   Critical thinking

What are your reactions to this sort of science, where researchers are engaged in openly political terms, righting perceived wrongs or else empowering others to change the healthcare world?

As this answer is based on your own observation, there is no outline answer at the end of the chapter.

Having formulated your reflections on research paradigms, turn back now to Table 3.1 in Chapter 3. There you will see described different levels of reasoning. Absolute reasoning associated with research paradigms might be to conclude that there is only one sort of 'proper research'. You might fiercely argue this against all comers, but are there any advantages in linking paradigms of research to different contexts and care requirements?

As you think about the different paradigms, it might be tempting to conclude that you should favour a single paradigm. But to back oneself into a philosophical corner might not prove that helpful. Nurses have to work pragmatically and imaginatively with different sorts of knowledge and a range of evidence within healthcare. It is, then, arguably appropriate to adopt a 'horses for courses' attitude towards knowledge. Instead of arguing that one sort of knowledge is superior, it may be appropriate to venture that the key consideration is to what purpose the evidence is put. If we are currently concerned with an intervention and what works, it is likely that we will search for and evaluate knowledge from the positivist paradigm. We will use questions that are appropriate there, which work with the claims of the research (research design and rigour). If we are currently concerned with insights and understanding patients better, we might search for information from the naturalistic paradigm and might ask different questions again. If a convincing case has been made for change, and the improvement involves a shift in power, we might draw on research from the critical theory paradigm and perhaps engage in research ourselves as part of an action research group. The key point is that we think critically in different ways and to strategic purpose. There is no one-size-fits-all way of reasoning possible here.

Asking different questions of evidence

It would be extremely helpful if research authors confided, at the outset, the paradigm within which they have framed their work. In practice, though, this does not always happen. Authors working within the positivist paradigm rarely allude to the philosophy of science that underpins their work, instead moving straight to the design of the survey or experiment. Researchers working within the naturalistic and critical theory paradigms are likely to be more explicit about their philosophical premises, and may refer to a research approach that is clearly aligned to certain beliefs about the nature of knowledge and its role in healthcare. You get a clearer steer as regards the basis on which they are presenting data and findings to you.

Activity 8.6 Group-working

To help you to test out my assertions above, arrange with your fellow students to each secure a research paper on an agreed theme (something of common interest to you all). Next, read your chosen paper, highlighting any passages of work that you think indicate the paradigm within which the work was conceived. Clues may be a focus on empirical data, traits, measurement, experimentation, and very detailed control measures in the research design, within positivist research. Clues to research conducted within the naturalistic paradigm include reference to research approaches used there, phenomenology, grounded theory, much ethnography, and – quite frequently – case study research. There is an emphasis on natural working environments, discovery, and insights into the experience of others. Clues to research conducted within the critical theory paradigm are terms such as 'feminist research' or 'Marxist research', and perhaps the use of 'action research' – work designed to produce rather than investigate change.

Next, summarise your paper to your fellow students, then discuss which paradigm you think it originated from and what that might mean for its contribution to nursing practice.

As this answer is based on your own observation, there is no outline answer at the end of the chapter.

Questions in the positivist paradigm

Where it is concluded that evidence has been produced within the positivist paradigm, a new group of questions becomes important (Edmonds and Kennedy, 2016). The first of these relates to the design of the research, and whether it has set out a clear question or hypothesis (a statement regarding what will or will not be the case). The research has to be clearly structured, and needs to state precisely which population of people it relates to and what the sample is. The way in which the sample was selected is important in this paradigm because the sample is sometimes argued to represent the population as a whole. The reader has to be convinced that the sample constitutes a reasonable proportion of the population concerned and matches its key features (e.g. age distribution, gender, health circumstances). Statistical guidance is usually sought as regards what represents an adequate sample, and beyond that a satisfactory return rate for questionnaires if a survey is used. Consideration of the population and sample size, the make-up of the sample, and whether it is representative of the population affect study *validity*. The research is valid if it addresses the research intention set and includes relevant and large enough samples of research subjects (people) or clinical circumstances. Small and unrepresentative samples of people can all undermine the validity of the research.

A second concern within positivist paradigm research is *reliability* (Edmonds and Kennedy, 2016) – whether, using the same data-gathering methods and the same research design, similar results could be obtained at a later date. Of course, when dealing with human beings, reliability could prove to be a problem. Positivist paradigm research works well where individuals behave or comment according to trait (i.e. consistently, indicative of their stable attitudes and values), but it is less reliable if people change their responses or behaviours dependent on circumstance (e.g. meeting a currently felt need). If people changed their mind frequently and behaved inconsistently, it would be difficult to judge whether the research was reliable.

I asked Stewart to summarise why positivist paradigm researchers were so interested in things such as validity and reliability. This is what he – quite reasonably – said:

> *Well, the research is about judging something, isn't it? And if you're going to claim that something is or is not proven, then you have to be sure that all your methods are well organised, that the work focuses on exactly the right thing. You have to be sure that others could repeat your work, to check that they got similar results.*

A further legitimate question regarding positivist paradigm research is that of bias. Has the researcher in some way, wittingly or otherwise, shaped the evidence so that it is not representative of reality (e.g. by using leading questions)? Has the researcher failed to resist the undue shaping of evidence by people or factors not anticipated in the research? Positivist paradigm researchers are keen to control for bias and to limit the risk that external factors in some way shape the data in ways that undermine subsequent claims about them.

Questions in the naturalistic paradigm

The critical questions to be asked of evidence stemming from the naturalistic paradigm are different and much more about comparing the researcher's account against your own experience of phenomena. This is because the world is conceived of more in terms of perception and experience. Everyone interprets their experiences and creates their own reality – their own account of what is really happening. So, for example, five people may visit the dentist and have treatment, but the experience and the meaning of these visits will depend as much on their perceptions of dentistry. The emphasis here is on the perceptual world, that which is negotiated and even co-created. Think, for example, about the meaning of old age: it is more than a physiological change; it is a complex experience.

Researchers working in this paradigm are not claiming to present a demonstrable truth that can be tested again and again, but a representation of what they have seen, heard and interpreted. Typically, the researcher deals with field observations and open-question interview responses, necessitating the presentation of possible themes, as well as that which might convey what has been experienced. The researcher cannot avoid using their own experiences to help make sense of what was said or witnessed. Because researchers are working with interpretations, it is accepted that what the researcher produces is at least in part a construction, something inherently shaped by the way in which information is collated and themes are represented. It is acknowledged that the researcher cannot but interpret and influence matters (e.g. through the line of questions that they pursue). To illustrate, a researcher exploring perceptions of visits to the dentist first collects the accounts of individuals who have been through this experience. The research interviews have not been rigidly constrained by set questions. Researchers follow lines of enquiry, those that help to clarify their opening ideas gleaned from past interviews. In explaining this (the audit trail), the researcher asks the reader to determine whether the research findings still seem trustworthy and valuable, as they return to the experience in question themselves. This might mean that you, as the reader, think again about what patients tell you, and it might guide some additional questions that you pose to them.

Remember that here, the concern is with the insight and understanding of a phenomenon, not with predicting what will happen in the future. So, the first question you should consider asking is whether or not there is a clear audit trail that describes how data were collected and analysed. Was this by interview or by observation, and in what order? How were the themes reported in the research arrived at? While all researchers need to describe the research design and steps taken, audit trailing is especially important in this paradigm. This is because the researcher presents their own 'take on reality'. Even if the researcher has laid out an adequate audit trail of their work, you might still question whether they have adequately considered all of the possible interpretations of the chosen phenomenon. Your test in this regard is whether something that seems important – from your own experience – has been considered. In this paradigm, the researchers believe that the world has potentially infinite experiences, interpretations and perceptions to report. They claim to capture some of these and invite your comparison from personal and professional experience. So, research evidence here might seem incomplete; it might miss something that you believe is important, especially in your practice context. Now the practice utility test is about completeness and fit of research design and evidence to clinical circumstances and needs. You are at liberty to observe, 'Ah, but have you thought about …?' or, 'In this context, patients are usually more concerned about …' As a reader of this sort of research, you are invited to think again, to focus afresh upon the phenomena in question. I tested this idea out with Raymet, asking her about audit trailing and why this was important in naturalistic paradigm research:

> *I think it's because researchers here accept that a lot of the important things which nurses are interested in cannot be proven, they cannot easily be measured. After all, being ill is extremely personal. Because of that, the researcher has to access the patient's experiences, which means they have to use a mix of questions, they need to find ways to relate to the patient. So, when I come to judge this research, I want to know about how they did that. I can then say, given my personal experience of illness or patients in the past, this does or doesn't sound convincing.*

As Raymet suggests, as well as asking questions about the audit trail, whether or not it was clear how the researchers proceeded, you also need to ask a question about authenticity: 'Given what I already know about this practice, do these findings seem credible?' (Holloway and Galvin, 2016). Of course, experiences elsewhere might not accord with your personal experience. They might be quite unique to another group of patients or practitioners. But if the research evidence is to be transferable, this concern with authentic, recognisable experience remains important. Quite a lot of naturalistic paradigm research evidence falters at this point. Human experience is contextual; it operates within a particular healthcare system. It may be authentic to local contexts, but it might not be transferable.

Questions in the critical theory paradigm

As critical theory research is polemical, consciously political, the first questions to ask here are: Are the researchers' premises about the need, problem or opportunity set out at the start? What is the research meant to correct or achieve? Honest critical theory paradigm research acknowledges from the outset what has framed and directed the research. The critical theory researcher would point out that truth is always contested, that the definition of what is happening is fought over. So, every position is in some sense partial, and reality is defined in terms favourable to the group holding power. However, they concede a responsibility to set out their alternative truth, what they wish to challenge. Having ascertained that the researchers' premises and assumptions are clear, the critical analysis of evidence moves to an audit trail, as above. How was the research conducted? Were the procedures here conducted in accord with the stated purpose of the research and the values of the researchers?

I discussed *action research*, a common method used within critical theory paradigm research, with Gina. She had seen action research under way in a clinic where she had recently been on practice placement. The research was all about developing a more consultative clinic, one that facilitated screening of sexually transmitted infections and contacts that the patient may have had. The researchers had stated that they felt the practitioners there were disempowered, being set targets and standards for the tracing of contacts, but with little help given on how to create an atmosphere more conducive to screening and tracing work. The researchers negotiated a series of activities, first to help the staff examine their concerns and needs, as well as the training that they might require. A second round of activity explored with them their values and attitudes towards risk and patient needs. Patients sought a degree of privacy, but the staff too needed to minimise risk for others, so work centred on facilitating responsibility in the patients. Gina observed:

> *It was egalitarian research; it did attend to staff needs and concerns, but it didn't lose sight of responsibility. Staff did have a duty of care to individual patients and they did have a public health responsibility too. So, in that sense, what the researchers did hold true to their stated values and goals without alienating the managers who had set targets in the first place. It was about how to work better.*

Reviewing critical theory paradigm research, then, is different to that linked to the naturalistic paradigm (which focuses on authenticity of the account) and radically different to that of the positivist paradigm (with its emphasis on reliability and validity). Here, the researcher acknowledges what they consider inequitable, unjust and problematic, as well as describing often collaborative research fieldwork designed to put things right. This has the propensity to make you think about your beliefs and values. Was this endeavour necessary? Do I share the beliefs and concerns of the researcher, and do I believe that their research aids in improving matters? In this paradigm, research does not stand aloof from politics and ideological debates; it drives straight in and provokes questions about the worthiness, the necessity, of particular healthcare.

The nature of evidence-based practice

The discussions above illustrate why research evidence is by no means a simple thing; it comes in many different forms and has been conceived of in different ways. You will need to reason at a high level (see Table 3.1 in Chapter 3) to do justice to a discussion of different sorts of research evidence. The purpose of research may be quite different, depending on how the research was conceived and where the information came from. For example, much research evidence within the naturalistic paradigm has been gathered to facilitate reflection. It raises questions such as 'Have you thought about this?' and 'Does this happen where you work?' Evidence associated with the positivist paradigm may contest current treatment or care; it might suggest what else works better, and the implicit questions are, then, 'Should we do something different?' and 'Should we continue doing this now?'

Evidence associated with the critical theory paradigm relates specifically to attitudes and values, the agendas and beliefs that might shape healthcare. Accepting the complexity of this, the questions posed, suggests that evidence-based practice will not be a one-size-fits-all matter either. Evidence-based practice may consist of changed care because a critical mass of what works, as well as knowledge about what is safe and critical to the improvement of the patient's condition, has accrued.

Evidence from the positivist paradigm is drawn upon, especially where that also accommodates consideration of the costs of healthcare. But evidence-based practice might also involve different ways to conceive of care partnerships, ways of working that show greater sensitivity to the needs of others. Evidence from the naturalistic or critical theory paradigms might be important here. Improvement in nursing care is still the central concern, but it is associated with different things, such as sensitivity, attuning care to patient requirements.

Successful evidence-based practice is, then, that which works with the strengths of different sorts of evidence, provided in association with different paradigms. There is recognition of the limitations of evidence, as well as what may be claimed about it. Nurses and other practitioners realise that evidence still requires interpretation and decisions about where and how best to use it. Evidence cannot substitute for clinical judgement and critical thinking. They need to be combined with these, and to strategic purpose.

Fundamental challenges usually remain:

- Have we got enough evidence?
- Does it all point in the same direction and suggest broadly the same things?
- Have we got a mix of evidence that attends to the aspects of care, what works, what is safe, and what reassures the patient?
- Is the evidence usable?

Chapter summary

You have now reached the end of Chapter 8 and your exploration of a particular sort of critical thinking, that which applies to evidence and its application in practice. Evidence is one of the key knowledge bases on which nurses draw. It is extremely important and yet hotly contested. If you are to critically examine evidence, it is necessary to understand what sorts of evidence there are, how these are related to paradigms of knowledge, and which questions are appropriate to employ there.

In this chapter, you have explored why both theory and research evidence might have to pass a utility test. Then you have explored different conceptions of evidence. To make sense of sometimes fiercely contested debates on evidence-based practice, you have looked at three paradigms, each of which shapes the ways in which people think about knowledge and conceive of evidence. Asking the right questions of evidence starts with an understanding of paradigms and remains mindful of practice utility, what works in a given clinical context.

Activities: brief outline answers

Activity 8.1 Reflection (page 129)

It seems odd to imagine a course dominated either by practice or theory – the challenge has always been to meld the two. Theory can help shape practice with new ideas and values, but few imagine theory entirely complete. In the past, practice was dominant and nurses learned to nurse through and apprenticeship. While some might feel nostalgic about those days, it seems doubtful that this form of learning would be equal to the complexity of care work today. Nurses have to think creatively, so we must speculate, theorise and debate, even if the subject matter does not entirely fit current practice. This process is taxing as nursing can seem impossibly complex, with a theory–practice gap questioning all that we strive for. My recommendation is to remember that not all theory or research serves practice; there is nursing beyond the bedside. However, to that I would add: do not be afraid to interrogate the seemingly fanciful; we need to imagine futures while acknowledging where we start from now.

Further reading

Linsley, P., Kane, R. and Barker, J. (2019) *Evidence-Based Practice for Nurses and Healthcare Professionals*, 4th edition. London: SAGE.

The authors provide a methodical review of how to evaluate evidence and then contemplate the best ways to improve practice. The book offers activities much like this one, so the style should seem familiar. Authors offer a range of competing perspectives on research and evidence, but this is a cogent and well-articulated one.

Useful websites

http://consumers.cochrane.org

The Cochrane Consumer Network is an offshoot of the original Cochrane Collaboration and is designed to help members of the general public become involved in the evaluation of healthcare evidence and the systematic reviews that the Cochrane Collaboration publishes. There is interesting video footage of consumers' views on this subject, as well as guidance on how members of the public can access research evidence, working through the complex terminology there.

www.cochrane.org/about-us

The Cochrane Collaboration provides an extensive collection of systematic reviews of research evidence and a free-to-access handbook on how to plan these, ensuring a rigorous evaluation process. Systematic reviews are rigorous methodological interrogations of intervention research that are usually associated with what effects an intervention has.

Chapter 9   Writing the analytical essay

Chapter aims

After reading this chapter, you will be able to:

- determine clearly the purpose of the analytical essays you write;
- identify the cases presented by others and what you will deliberate upon;
- adopt a clear position on the case within your analytical essay;
- select relevant evidence and link this to arguments within your written work;
- demonstrate more speculative and scholarly ways of writing in your essays;
- prepare conclusions that both sum up previous texts and demonstrate what you deduce from them.

Introduction

Throughout your nursing career, writing essays will be part of the work required to demonstrate progress. There is little room for absolute thinking, where you advocate only one cause, where you neglect the options, opinions and debates that encircle modern nursing practice. You will need to write in a critical way.

This chapter combines my previous teaching on critical thinking and writing, and applies it to analytical essays. I remind you of some of the characteristics of more critical thinking that you first met in Table 3.1 in Chapter 3. I consider the purposes to which the analytical essay is put, and highlight the importance of clearly establishing your position before you start writing. I review how best to discriminate what should be included in the essay, and then the use of arguments that demonstrate your ability to weigh the merits and limitations of a case. I revisit how best to sum up the essay within the conclusion, and make the point that success here consists of much more than simply repeating what has been presented earlier in the paper.

The purpose of analytical essays

Analytical essays are set for different purposes. The first of these is to test your understanding of a given subject and your ability to make a series of well-informed judgements about it (the evaluative essay). Such essays are frequently set as a review of the literature, research reports or healthcare policies. Examiners wish to understand whether you have a clear grasp of what others have argued, and whether you have developed a clear perspective of your own. Evaluative essays are sometimes set early on within a course to check your grasp of key concepts. If you do not understand these concepts, you may find subsequent learning more difficult, and it will be hard for teachers to build on your raft of existing knowledge.

The second purpose of the analytical essay is to move forward from this, to assess your strategic thinking: What would you do next, and why? A strategic essay might set you a clinical problem or invite you to weigh conflicting demands before advocating your own best course of action. It may test your ability to make choices and the ordering of work in a logical sequence.

The third purpose is to test your ability to confront conundrums or to examine professional ethos (the philosophical essay). Essays of these kind often test your highest-level reasoning skills (see Table 3.1 in Chapter 3) because you have to ruminate on values, attitudes, priorities and principles in a way that shows you are thinking about care as a whole (i.e. in metacognition). Sometimes there is no straightforward answer and no neat solution, and the nurse has to manage a situation as it is. Papers about ethical dilemmas may be of this kind.

Activity 9.1   Critical thinking

Below are some essay assignment questions or instructions. Decide which purpose each of these questions serves.

1. The attached case study describes the experiences of Avril, a 35-year-old woman with learning difficulties. She lives within a community home with five other residents. Read the account of Avril's relationship with

(Continued)

(Continued)

    Tony, another resident, and then critically discuss the challenges that arise in association with contraception here.

2. 'Nurses are necessarily interpreters of healthcare policies.' With reference to a policy of your own choosing, critically discuss whether you support this statement. Remember to back up your points with reference to the literature and/or observations from practice.

3. As part of a new initiative to engage the public in strategic healthcare planning, four ex-patients have become consultants to your nursing team. How will you work with them to enhance the services delivered to patients? Make sure that you refer to theories of leadership and change agency taught during your course.

My answers to this activity are given at the end of the chapter.

The case and the position taken

Having established the purpose of the forthcoming essay (what the question asks), our next job is to determine what position we take and what case will be considered. The two are not necessarily the same. A case might be stated as part of the question and you are asked to examine it. Question 2 in Activity 9.1 does just that; the case is stated briefly, simply, that nurses are interpreters of healthcare policies. You present questions and arguments that explain your position on this given case. In other instances, you make the opening case in the essay and back this up with arguments. Under examination conditions, being clear about the case and your position is critical. However, we are often so keen to make the best use of the time available that we set to quickly, writing down points that are confused. We seem unsure about the case and indecisive about our position. Yet we know that by the end of the essay, our position has to be very clear. For example, relating to Activity 9.1, we might decide that we support the statement in question 2 about nurses interpreting policy, but with certain caveats. There are some restrictions because nurses must simultaneously apply several policies and each demands priority attention (what you have learned about assessing information utility in Chapter 8 will be relevant here). You might support the case that nurses interpret policy, but your position is a qualified one. It is vital, then, before you write, even in an examination, to pause and consider what your position will be. If you have the chance to make a case of your own, what will that be?

Activity 9.2   Reflection

Stewart confided in me that he did not always clarify his position before writing essays. He feared that examiners might judge him negatively if his perspective did not mirror theirs. He tried to write an answer that he hoped might please the examiner.

Reflect now on whether this worry has affected you too. Is it as important a problem as not knowing what your position is in the first place? Once you have done this, look back at Table 3.1 in Chapter 3 to remind yourself that in academic settings, the last thing that assessors expect is for you to present an absolute case, one which does not consider other possibilities. There is often no single right answer, only ones that have a clearer reasoning audit trail within them.

As this answer is based on your own observation, there is no outline answer at the end of the chapter.

Establishing your position is important. This is because it will determine what arguments you make within the essay and what evidence you draw on. Some positions require a great deal of evidence to support them, reflecting the complexity and ambiguities of nursing care. If we continue with the above example, we would need to identify circumstances where:

- we definitely should interpret the chosen policy;
- there is more limited scope to interpret the policy;
- factors combine to severely restrict our ability to interpret the policy.

On balance, if we support the case, the first group of these factors should predominate. Showing that other factors intervene, though, and that there are caveats to consider, demonstrates that our judgement is not rash. In an essay such as this, we might draw on evidence from the literature that is connected to local protocols and standard care pathways, as well as observations from practice and discussions with fellow students who have managed policy implementation in the past.

Activity 9.3 Critical thinking

What sort of brief answer plan might you use in an examination situation to help you prepare an answer that demonstrates your position clearly in response to a question? Jot down an idea or two, perhaps describing a plan that you use now.

My suggested plan is given at the end of the chapter.

Arguments and evidence

We have already seen in Chapter 3 that an essay is composed of a series of sections (introduction, main text, conclusion), which are in turn made up of a sequence of paragraphs, within which we advance our arguments. Coherent essays have arguments that fit with the position being defended and they lead appropriately to the conclusion. In Chapter 7, I clarified what formal arguments look like; they usually include the word 'because', which helps to link the case to the underpinning premises. In essays, however, not every one of your arguments will be constituted that formally. Sometimes you will present opinions or perspectives. Your arguments, though, will still need to be supported by evidence.

We might arrange the essay in several ways; for example, reviewing the alternative positions that might be adopted with regard to nurses' interpretation of healthcare policy, before revealing the position that evidence seems to support. Alternatively, our position may seem so strong that we state this at the outset, and then lead the reader through stepwise arguments that demonstrate its power. A committed stance of this kind is not simply absolute thinking. The case is backed up by a series of carefully considered arguments in support of it. Some evidence is adopted, and other evidence is challenged as being unclear, poorly articulated or perhaps less relevant to the context in hand. The assessor is left in no doubt that you have pondered your answer with care.

It is disempowering to feel that the only arguments which can fairly be advanced in an essay are those that are supported within the literature. This appears to suggest that the only valid form of knowledge is that which has been published. In truth, a significant amount of evidence remains unpublished, and this includes some research findings, audits of practice and observations made in practice. There are different sorts of evidence (Whitman et al., 2017; see also Chapter 8). Before you can couple evidence with your chosen arguments, you need to ascertain how powerful the evidence is and whether it clearly supports the point that you wish to make. A poorly selected piece of evidence can undermine your essay.

Activity 9.4   Critical thinking

Look at the following examples of evidence coupled with arguments that you might include within an essay on interpreting local healthcare policy. Determine whether you think the evidence supports the chosen argument. Then decide whether the pairings seem convincing to you.

1. *The argument:* Nurses are confident enough to examine policies critically because they are acquainted with the legal, ethical and practical constraints that apply to it.

The evidence: Nurse researchers report in a journal article their grounded theory research, which included interviews with and observations of nurses in practice. The research articulates how nurses reason care in action, including that pertaining to policy implementation.

2. *The argument*: Nurses have advanced some areas of the chosen policy and delayed others, acknowledging that patients are ill-equipped to partner every aspect of care.

   The evidence: A series of audit case studies have been compiled locally that itemise which elements of shared decision-making patients expect to engage in and which they have misgivings about.

3. *The argument*: Nurses have limits set on policy interpretation because older policies are still in place and have not yet been updated to help facilitate the proposed way forward.

   The evidence: Two standard care pathways in operation in local clinical areas are cited as examples of situations where practitioners sometimes express their frustration.

My reflections are given at the end of the chapter.

Deciding which arguments and evidence make it into your essay is critical. You may have previously encountered essay feedback where the tutor has told you that your account was 'too superficial'. You are likely to be guilty of this if you try to include too many arguments and pieces of evidence. Evidence needs to be introduced and you need to make points about it. The exasperated assessor might observe, 'You seem to record everyone else's opinion but not arrive at a perspective of your own!' This is often a problem where you are not thinking critically enough, showing due regard to the specific circumstances alluded to within the essay question, or else you have not applied your points to a care location. Remember that higher-order critical reasoning shows greater precision; it is contextualised as well as inquisitive. Fewer carefully chosen arguments, as well as being more selective about what evidence you use to support them, will often stand your work in good stead.

Speculating successfully

Something that students find very difficult to achieve within an essay is speculation. If arguments are founded upon evidence, and evidence is contradictory or even absent, how do we proceed? We are left to rehearse what could be happening or what might be done next. We need to identify what can be suggested, whether that is within the literature or as part of clinical experience. We also need to imagine the future, how services might change, what patient needs could be, and how we might work better with relatives.

Speculation is an important part of higher-level critical thinking. Nursing practice needs nurses who are confident and willing to speculate, to imagine what might be the case, what could be required. Failing to ask the right questions often means that opportunities for improvements in practice are lost. In Table 3.1 in Chapter 3, the highest level of critical thinking is demonstrated by asking imaginative questions in care situations.

To speculate with confidence, we need to use terms which signal to the reader that we have moved into speculative mode. If we signal these matters clearly and then write in a measured way about the subject (i.e. without stating what we think is 'obvious' or 'self-evident', or what 'naturally follows'), we will be taking the reader along with us, reasoning at our side.

The following words and short phrases all signal that we are speculating:

- *Notionally*: This suggests that we are considering an embryonic idea – one still in development. For example: 'Notionally, nurses do more to interpret policies than they realise. Even simple care involves interpreting what equals quality.'
- *Arguably*: This is used to suggest that the point is sufficiently clear and coherent to constitute an argument, but it is one we are still considering. For example: 'Nurses' frustration with policy is arguably to do with constraints on professional freedom.'
- *We might speculate*: This is a tentative way of putting things, suggesting an area of enquiry or a line of reasoning. For example: 'We might speculate that while standard care plans save nurses' time, they also limit thinking.'
- *A number of possibilities present*: This sets out possible explanations. For example: 'A number of possibilities present that: first, colleagues insist on writing their own policies; second, they form alliances with policymakers; and third, they lament change but persevere with their instructions.'
- *It would be possible to suggest*: This hints that what is written about next has some credibility. For example: 'It would be possible to suggest that nurses are shaping the policies which matter – those that determine the experience of care.'
- *Conceivably*: This suggests something that could be considered but might not be the easiest explanation. For example: 'Conceivably, nurse entrepreneurs are those who see policy as a lever. They use it to achieve desirable ends.'

Activity 9.5   Reflection

Look back over some past essays and note whether you used any of the above words or phrases to indicate that you were speculating. Did you use the words in the right way?

As this answer is based on your own observation, there is no outline answer at the end of the chapter.

Reaching successful conclusions

A large majority of analytical essays written by students describe what has gone before within the essay, but without necessarily demonstrating a conclusion. To use a simple analogy, we describe a journey made (we spent three hours on the train). What is usually required within an analytical essay is to determine the significance of that journey. We can illustrate this by referring to the three purposes of analytical essays described earlier:

- *Evaluative*: The journey was arduous, took longer than expected, and prompted us to reconsider the advantages of using public transport in the future.
- *Strategic*: There remain opportunities to improve upon the journey, at least with regard to the time taken. Weekday public transport schedules are better.
- *Philosophical*: Travelling by public transport had the advantage of reducing our carbon footprint. Had we driven there, the environmental penalty would have been higher.

A successful conclusion, then, must capture the account of what has been written so far (the journey) but must also include a deduction. We have to make clear what matters seem settled and what remain open at the end of the essay. Contrary to what some students think, it is not always true that we need to have 'nailed our colours to the mast', either wholeheartedly adopting or rejecting the case presented to us in a question. We do, however, need to have clarified our position: 'The case seems supportable to this extent, but what we need to ascertain further is XYZ.'

In the following example of a concluding paragraph relating to the essay on policy interpretation, there is a clear indication of the author's resting position at the end. Notice how the author refers back to the case that has already been introduced at the start of the essay:

> *At the start of this paper, I introduced the case that nurses do interpret policies, but cautioned that their success in this is affected by factors that limit their freedom to proceed at will. The paper highlights that pressure of time and the need to serve a public, as well as individual patients, to work effectively in teams and to attend to employer agendas, all shape the interpretation of healthcare policy. My chosen policy (rehabilitation) espouses a philosophy of cooperation and consultation. Nurses might wish to interpret this policy as an opportunity to deliver individualised care, but they do not always have the scope to proceed in that way. Instead, the need to ration their expertise and attention serves to contain just how much consultation they engage in.*

In this conclusion, the journey is summed up quickly in the sentence describing what limits nurses' opportunities to interpret policy. The telling point arrives at the end, where it is explained that the nurse might wish to interpret policy in a particular way (as individualised care), but that care is necessarily rationed. The nurse does a little for the many and not as much as might be wished for the few. The author defends the opening case.

Drafting the essay and checking it

Students vary in their preferred ways of writing and editing. Having prepared an outline plan that signals the key sections of the paper, the arguments and evidence that will appear in each, the case that will be considered and the position adopted, some quickly set down a first draft. Students may have checked that they remain within the word counts they have allocated for each section, but they will leave any references, tables and quotes to be added later. The first goal for such students is to get work down on paper that captures their understanding of the subject and which represents their position regarding it. Other students move much more incrementally, carefully crafting each section and adding embellishments as they go. However you proceed, though, checking the clarity and coherence of what has been written remains a responsibility.

I asked the four case study nursing students about their essay drafting and reviewing processes:

Gina: If you write a 'rough' draft of your essay in one sitting, you have the advantage that you don't pause to fret over doubts as you go. Afterwards, though, you need to check whether the arguments stacked up.

Fatima: I work with my plan, especially as regards the word allowance. If one section seems tight and I need to include more words than I hoped, I stop right then and ask whether I'm trying to include too much.

Raymet: I write first draft essays in the morning and then talk the content of my essay through with a friend. I explain what I am arguing. If they seem clear about my thoughts, even if they don't agree with my position, I feel encouraged.

Stewart: Writing for me is private, but I always leave several days to complete an edit. My later essays have been better for that.

I agree with Gina that doubts can creep in as you write. Sometimes work grinds to a halt if you do not write a little more quickly and freely in the first instance. There is something to be said, then, for writing a first complete but more rudimentary draft. It probably captures your position most cleanly, provided that you have allocated enough thinking time before starting work.

Fatima's approach is much more 'sculpted'. The work proceeds in sections and each is 'got right' before the next is attempted. The approach does produce work that has well-balanced sections, spreading the allocation of words allowed. Students sometimes discover their position shifting a little as they write in this way. It is then necessary to check what is claimed in the introduction – do you still support that?

I especially support Raymet's strategy of summarising a first draft essay. Notice that Raymet sticks to her guns once she has identified what her position will be. This is commendable, provided you have heard and considered the questions and challenges posed by others. Your friend might not have read what you have or attended the lectures that you did, so their position on a subject cannot be yours. Against that, naive questions and thoughtful challenges from reviewers are valuable, as you might well have missed something. To avoid charges of academic collusion and dishonesty, resist the temptation to ask them to edit your essay. This should remain your own work.

If you have left insufficient time to review work, or are preparing several papers in quick succession, essay editing can seem a bit of a chore. It is tempting to submit the work and hope. Time spent checking, however, is beneficial in several ways. You can:

- conduct the spelling, syntax and other presentational checks;
- ensure that the work answers the question or attends to the task set;
- assure yourself that a case has been made – one that is supported, rejected or seen as conditional within the conclusion.

Before closing this chapter, I want to remind you of the importance of representing your sources (citing where they come from) and using quotes in a clear and consistent way. I introduced the risks of plagiarism in Chapter 3, but your last checks on the essay that you have prepared can help you to avoid unwittingly committing plagiarism. Remember that if in doubt, it is always better to ask a tutor about your work, whether a particular passage avoids plagiarism. Once the work is submitted, you are attesting that what you have provided includes clear attribution of all sources. The most common cases of plagiarism investigated are those associated with inadequate **citation** and failing to represent the exact words of others accurately using quotation marks (Price, 2014).

Citing others' work

Remember that it is your responsibility to adequately represent where information has come from, irrespective of whether it is published or unpublished, whether it comes from a website or a book/journal, or whether the work is that of your tutor, senior colleagues at work or your employer (Price, 2014). Sources may be primary (where the information is first presented) or secondary (where the original information is summarised by another). It is usually best to represent the original reference where available, by indicating the author(s) name and the year of publication within your text, next to the point that they make. If in doubt, repeat that citation in more than one place – saying that you cited the source three pages ago is not sufficient. If you do use a secondary source, it is important to represent both sources in a bracket, (author A cited in author B's work, and date). Sometimes students rely quite heavily on a secondary author because they summarise points rather well. You would, though, plagiarise that second author's work if you used their words without clear citation in your text and without the use of quotation marks. Secondary authors' words are not a substitute for your own critique.

As I indicated in Chapter 3, it is necessary to find a balance of others' words and your own reasoning within an essay. A work full of quotes and little analysis of your own will not win you plaudits. Sometimes then it is necessary to paraphrase the work of another author, perhaps because you wish to express their point rather more succinctly, or to quickly connect it to arguments made by other authors. Students sometimes become confused about paraphrasing, the process of summarising others' arguments in your own words. If you use their exact words, this represents a quote, so check that you have enclosed the passage in quotation marks and cited the source, as above. If you have changed their words to your own, then you still need to cite the source. The fact that you have added an interpretation or a new combination of words does not absolve you from that responsibility. Just how many words need to be changed for a paraphrase not to require quotation marks is sometimes debated (Price, 2014). However, I suggest that you create brand new sentences, and that you avoid passages of words which the other author used. Clearly, if they present a key term (e.g. 'person-centred history-taking'), that has to be included. But be bold – translate what they say into something that is your own. Here is one last illustration:

> *Original text passage:* Patient anxiety is not only associated with the threat posed (e.g. an operation, a clinical procedure), but with the patient's predisposition to be fearful. The human brain processes potential threat and potential pleasure within the amygdala. In some instances, life experiences may predispose the individual to anticipate threat more than pleasure.

> *Adequate paraphrase:* Patients are sometimes predisposed to identify threat within a wide variety of situations met. Irrespective of how painful or risky a treatment is (actual threat), they can still be fearful (surname of original author and date).

Once you have completed the last citation and quotation requirements, check that all your references appear in the list at the end of your work, and that the details included in the text (surname and date) match that which is included in your reference list.

Chapter summary

Each individual essay is a work that operates in context, attending to the question or task set. Even though this is an academic work, it still expresses your preferred ways of working. You are the person who drafts the work and you write in a way that enables you to present scripts on time. There are, however, certain features of good analytical essay-writing that show your critical thinking at work. You need to be very clear about the purpose of the essay and to write in the appropriate way. Are you going to evaluate or philosophise, for example? You need to determine what case is being discussed and what position you take on it. In some instances, an examiner will set the case by making an assertion that you are invited to evaluate. In other instances, you select a case of your own – one that you will defend using arguments and evidence as your essay unfolds. Good analytical essay-writing includes sufficient arguments and pieces of evidence to make a clear case. There is a balance struck between analytical writing (what you think) and descriptive writing (what you report). Where the debate remains open and the best way forward is still to be discovered, you will make selective use of more speculative forms of writing. Conclusions are arranged in such a way that they do more than describe what has been discussed in the text. They indicate where your reasoning has led. All of this is improved where you allocate sufficient time to editing your own work.

Activities: brief outline answers

Activity 9.1 Critical thinking (page 143)

1. This is a tricky one. There are ethical and philosophical issues at stake here surrounding human and reproductive rights, so the essay has a philosophical purpose. It is strategic too, though, as challenges in this instance seem to pose the question 'What will you do next?' In these instances, the clues to what may be required often exist in the case study.

2. The purpose here is evaluative. The opening assertion, about nurses interpreting policy, makes this clear. Do you support this case?

3. The purpose here is strategic. The essay requires you to write about how you might involve lay consultants in the business of care delivery.

Activity 9.3 Critical thinking (page 144)

One plan that I have found workable is as follows:

*   Essay purpose: what is asked of me?

*   Case made: mine or the examiner's (name it)?

*   My position: for or against the case, caveats noted.

*   Section 1: introduction and signposting.

*   Section 2: main body.

*   Key arguments and paired evidence (argument 1, evidence; argument 2, evidence; etc.).

*   Section 3: conclusions.

Activity 9.4 Critical thinking (page 146)

Did you notice how some of the arguments were formally worded, including the word 'because'? It would be possible to debate these in philosophical terms if the premises were then spelled out.

The first argument is really about the potential of nurses to interpret policies because of what they consider as part of that process. The research evidence (grounded theory) illustrates how nurses do this. Whether nurses within your chosen context exhibit the same potential may be debatable.

The second argument is about nurses' judgement. The claim is that policy is implemented to a degree, sometimes because patients are not ready to collaborate in care. In this instance, there is a very good fit of evidence – a local audit has determined what patients feel able to do. The argument is supported if the discussion is about a policy interpreted locally.

The third argument is about constraints. Not all policies are written so as to advance care together. Older policies (in this instance, standard care pathways) are working at odds with the new policy. Once again, the evidence seems a promising match, although it is not inconceivable that nurses might not find an adequate compromise between the old and new policies, and this could represent interpretation of policy.

Further reading

Greetham, B. (2018) *How to Write Better Essays,* 4th edition. London: Palgrave Macmillan.

I think that you should be a little cautious about 'quick fix' essay-writing guidance tomes, but Bryan Greetham's work has stood the test of time. It attends both to reasoning and essay structure, something that I advocate strongly in my own book. It is not a book written specifically for nurses, but the tenets of good practice are still liberally scattered throughout this text.

Wallace, M. and Wray, A. (2016) *Critical Reading and Writing for Postgraduates,* 3rd edition. London: SAGE.

While this book is firmly aimed at postgraduate students, a wide range of learners should still find it of value. Both undergraduate and postgraduate students are often asked to 'critically evaluate the literature', weighing up what the balance of literature offers as well as evaluating what individual authors claim. The case example of essay work within this chapter is firmly an applied subject, so you might find it useful to supplement reading where literature alone is the focus of attention.

Useful website

https://en.wikibooks.org/wiki/Writing_Better_University_Essays

This free-to-access e-book provides a good array of guidance on essay-writing in coursework and examination contexts. Although not specifically aimed at healthcare students, the guidance usually holds good as regards the principles of analytical writing. I liked the summary of common problems met with in essay-writing.

Chapter 10 Writing the reflective essay

NMC Standards of Proficiency for Registered Nurses

This chapter will address the following platforms and proficiencies:

Platform 1: Being an accountable professional

At the point of registration, the registered nurse will be able to:

1.3 Understand and apply the principles of courage, transparency and the professional duty of candour, recognising and reporting any situations, behaviours or errors that could result in poor care outcomes.

1.10 Demonstrate resilience and emotional intelligence and be capable of explaining the rationale that influences their judgments and decisions in routine, complex and challenging situations.

Chapter aims

After reading this chapter, you will be able to:

- identify the important tasks to be attended to when writing a reflective essay;
- discuss the functions of the reflective essay and how this affects its construction;
- explain clearly the purpose of reflective essays;
- demonstrate insights into the reporting of events, feelings, perceptions, perspectives, interpretations, conclusions, and planned next actions associated with reflection.

Introduction

It is in the nature of nursing that we need to reflect and be able to write reflectively. Nurses deal with human experience. There are sometimes no 'right solutions' in healthcare, only better reasoned courses of action, those founded to a significant extent upon reflection (Monrouxe and Rees, 2017). Much of what nurses currently aspire to in their work relies upon the adequate recognition of patients' experiences, as well as the ability to summarise and convey them to others (Price, 2019b). It is because nurses need to access their experience in a clear and consistent way, and because we need to understand the process of reviewing the same, that reflection and reflective writing are so important.

Reflection is also important if we are to manage successfully the stresses of nursing care (Steele, 2020). We must judge, for instance, the right level of closeness to maintain with patients, many of whom are distressingly sick. Nursing work is demanding, especially where we have discovered that we believe different things to other people, and where values might then clash. Nursing sometimes exposes us to conflict, so it is vital that we are able to make sense of events. We need to be aware of what we believe and value, as well as respecting the beliefs of others, if we are to practise well (Skela-Savič et al., 2017). Table 3.2 in Chapter 3 details the different expressions of reflective reasoning as you move from absolute thinking through transitional and contextual thinking and on to the deepest introspection within independent thinking.

In this chapter, I examine a series of key tasks associated with the business of writing reflectively, tasks linked to reflective writing coursework. Next, I give consideration to the reflective frameworks that you might be invited to use within your coursework. These vary by college and course, but are certain common principles. All of these frameworks ask you to attend to feelings, meanings and then actions. Finally, I turn to the different levels of critical reflection, first introduced in Table 3.2 in Chapter 3. In practice (and importantly for assessment), I argue that there are gradations of reflection, with levels reaching well beyond the description and summary of events.

Five key tasks of reflective writing

Irrespective of whether your reflective writing takes the form of a coursework essay, a report from a clinical practice placement, or practice reflections made for revalidation (NMC, 2019), there are five tasks that your work should attend to.

1. Representing enquiry

Reflection is a form of enquiry that sees you return to experience, delve into attitudes and values, or explore the possibilities of practice. As we have seen in Chapter 2, reflection may happen while you are in action (delivering care) or after action (when you take a retrospective view). In the first of these instances, your reflections are likely to be less well developed. You will need to show the reader how you are speculating about what is happening, something we touched on in Chapter 9. All reflective writing, however, needs to explain quickly the purpose and process of the enquiry in which you are engaged. Setting up these explanations at the start of your written work will help read-ers to review your work with greater insight into that achieved. As we will see below, you can only demonstrate higher-level reflective reasoning, contextual thinking, if there is a clear purpose or context to your writing.

Activity 10.1 Communication

I asked Fatima and Gina to share with me some of the opening paragraphs they have written at the start of reflective essays. Then I asked them to summarise these into a clear purpose and process for each. Their summaries are provided below. Read each of these and then prepare brief notes on why working on such summaries might improve your reflective writing.

Fatima: The purpose of this essay is to explore the ways in which I negotiated care with a family supporting a dying patient. To that end, I arrange my reflections using a series of headings, those first associated with my assumptions and perceptions of care needs, those I believed that the family held, and then the compromises that were agreed between us.

Gina: The purpose of this essay is to uncover some of the values, beliefs and aspirations that I hold with regard to holistic care. This work involved critical reflections regarding what each element of holistic care entails, and what I could reasonably deliver on. My reflections conclude with a summary of the discrepancies that remain, between what I believe I should deliver and what I succeed in assisting patients with.

As this answer is based on your own observation, there is no outline answer at the end of the chapter.

Imagine that Fatima or Gina simply launched into the description of a care episode. It would be difficult to determine what they were trying to understand from their experi-ence. The description of an episode alone does not signal what the focus of enquiry was. It is much better to start with a stated purpose that gives rigour to your reflective writing.

2. Distinguishing between facts, perspectives, perceptions, narratives and discourses

Reflective writing deals with facts (e.g. the dosage of a drug taken), but it also deals regularly with perspectives and perceptions. We need to show that we appreciate the dis-tinctions between these within our work. A perspective is something that sums up our position, values, aspirations and beliefs. It is closely associated with a disposition to think of things in an enduring way (Aleshire et al., 2019). For example, 'Care should be person-centred, working with the individual's needs' is an expression of a perspective. It is often used to describe what we think should be the case or what we think should happen. A perception, though, is much more fragile than this and describes the impressions that we take from incomplete or fragmentary experiences. 'Mrs Jones was upset; she searched for words to express all the worries that came with the diagnosis' is an example of a perception. We have no direct proof of what Mrs Jones felt, as she has not told us, but we infer things from that witnessed.

In some instances, you may have access to a patient or colleague narrative under development, the story that they use to explain what is happening and what they are trying to do. Narratives are a way of organising perceptions so that they make personal sense (Buckley et al., 2018). Where narratives are combined and perhaps shared with others to explain more complex interactions (e.g. the process of rehabilitating after an injury), we refer to *discourses*. Discourses capture the nature and purpose of activity, the bigger issues that are involved in healthcare (e.g. leadership, power, empowerment, therapy) (Vinson, 2016). Discourses frequently evaluate the activity undertaken, so a discourse might be about improvement or failure, success or confusion. They may be overtly political, relating to what the parties involved believe should happen.

Much of what we reflect upon in essays revolves around facts, perceptions and perspectives. A number of mistakes are easily possible as we draft our work:

- We may allow our perspective to dominate how we imagine others think or feel (they believe what I believe).
- We may infer perspectives held by others based on quite limited perceptions of what they do or say (we fill in the gaps).
- We may build a perspective based on a series of perceptions, each of which is reasonable in and of itself, but which become more suspect as we string them together.
- We muddle perception and fact, writing about perceptions as fact.

When you review the points above, you might note that many of these mistakes are associated with lower levels of reflective reasoning (see Table 3.2 in Chapter 3). Allowing your perspective to dominate how you imagine others think or feel is an absolute way of thinking. You have not imagined that there could be other perspectives to be taken into account. Deducing something from insufficient information suggests quite rudimentary transitional thinking. Reflection requires us to explore some more, to imagine issues and concerns, to conduct what I described as speculation within Chapter 9.

To write successfully, it is necessary to be clear about whether you are writing about a fact, a perspective, a perception, a narrative or a discourse. In many of the best reflective essays, nurses write about competing narratives or discourses, ways in which individuals and groups understand events. They speculate about the perceptions that others may have regarding the situation. Rather than close that debate, arguing that this or that is therefore the case, they acknowledge that the situation remains ambiguous and that further interpretation is needed. Here is a successful example from Gina's work on holistic care:

Spiritual care was challenging for me as I typically associated it with religious belief, and especially my religious beliefs. So, my default perspective was that to talk about spiritual care was to talk about how others live their religious convictions. It seemed apparent, though, that other people, including those who were not overtly religious, were also spiritual. This appeared to be associated with that which was aesthetic, beautiful, meaningful, especially as regards good living. I discovered that it was about that which made people feel dignified.

The key point here, then, is not to confuse the reader regarding what you are writing about. Distinguish clearly between terms such as 'perception' and 'perspective', and use these terms consistently.

3. Demonstrating insight

In many instances, reflective writing requires you to take a risk to share with the reader some insights into your beliefs, ways of thinking and operating. At best, these insights demonstrate your quizzical attitude towards practice. In Table 3.2 in Chapter 3, independent thinking (the highest standard of reflection), relating to the understanding of yourself, involves seeing experience as an opportunity to re-examine your own values, beliefs and attitudes. It can feel uncomfortable to write in this way, especially if you fear that the reader will condemn you for what you have not achieved. In a healthcare culture that expects excellence, it is more difficult to confide things about what seemed imperfect regarding your work.

To help you share insights more openly, it is worth checking with your tutor in advance that the essay is being assessed as evidence of continued learning and professional growth. Well-written assignment briefs should make this apparent from the outset. To confide that you have behaved in an unprofessional or illegal manner may still mean that the work triggers some form of sanction. The reflective essay is not a confessional that absolves you of all guilt for acts that have been dangerous or demeaning for patients.

The important point here is first to liaise with your tutor to check the purpose of the reflective essay set. Then, when it is clear that you should evaluate your own practice and reasoning, pick out what you have assumed, what requires further attention. The writing does not need to seem revelatory, to the extent that you will now completely change all that you do, but it should demonstrate a clearer understanding of what now seems problematic, incomplete, less sensitive, or perhaps what has been successful or effective.

Take a look now at a brief passage of my past reflective writing to see what I mean by demonstrating insight. I question my previous assumptions and think afresh about what that implies from the days when I ran altered body image workshops for patients dealing with chronic illnesses. Notice that I do not simply dismiss my past reasoning, but I do think that it needs to be refined. This is an entirely quizzical stance to take, and incidentally one that is important in professional revalidation as well (NMC, 2019):

Having explained to the patients ways in which body image could be expressed, I shifted from explaining terms to welcoming reflections from the group. I assumed, somewhat naively, that patients could, with gentle support, objectify the body, talking about it as something owned and separate from self. The body (as I had described it) was a home that they lived in, a resource that enabled them to express themselves. Incrementally, though, I realised that for some patients, the idea of body and self were not separate. The body was self, and therefore the illness seemed a direct assault on all that they stood for. They did not feel able to reason about their changed body until they had finished grieving for their lost health. A Muslim friend of mine explained that he saw his body as a temple where religious convictions were expressed. That idea was similar to mine, but he observed that those from other traditions and cultures might not think as he and I did. To see the body as something owned that we were responsible for was perhaps uncomfortable.

Significant implications followed from this. First, it would be harder to run group workshops for patients unless they first shared ways of thinking about the body (perhaps a cultural matter). Second, grieving for lost health might determine when the patient was ready to join a group. However efficient it might be to run rehabilitation groups, for some rehabilitation would need to be through one-to-one support and counselling.

My attitude is inquisitive, is it not? Notice too that the reflection spells out a 'so what' message. Simply put, it would be untenable to run all of my support through a group setting. Patients might not be ready for that. The deductions that I draw are about what seems workable in the future.

Activity 10.2   Reflection

Pause to write a short passage of reflective work where you question your own reasoning. Try to determine where you have thought too narrowly, a little naively or without reference to some important information.

As this answer is based on your own observation, there is no outline answer at the end of the chapter.

4. Respecting others

When writing reflectively, we run the risk of expressing prejudices, which demonstrates a disregard for others. This is not simply a matter of political correctness; *The Code* (NMC, 2018a) makes it very clear that we must have regard for the feelings and concerns of others and protect their human rights. It is necessary to write circumspectly and to consider carefully whether expressed attitudes might signal a disregard for patients or colleagues. This requirement relates not only to those of a different gender, age, colour, culture, religious background or sexual identity from your own, but to any with whom you have professional working relationships. Check therefore that what you include in your reflection demonstrates a respect for others. By all means, acknowledge difference – the diversity of human experience and need – but do not assume that your own perspectives on matters are inherently superior.

Activity 10.3   Critical thinking

Below are two service issues that might feature in a reflective practice essay. Make brief notes on why these issues require sensitivity when writing reflectively upon practice.

1. *Consumerism:* A patient and their family research the internet to back up claims regarding what they feel entitled to.

2. *Professional ideology and personal belief:* A patient consistently refuses regular analgesia when it is offered, stating that his religious faith requires him to tolerate a degree of pain.

My suggestions are offered at the end of the chapter.

5. Illustrating learning

Your reflective essay has one further function: to demonstrate your learning. If you write in a static way, about an unquestioned perspective or perceptions that seem set in stone, you are unlikely to have attended to the last of the five tasks – the illustration of learning. Good reflective writing takes the reader on a journey, from that which is shared at the start of the essay to that which is shared at the end. In this regard, reflective writing stands in sharp contrast to other forms of academic writing. In the analytical essay, the student often creates a case and then defends that using a series of arguments within the main text (see Chapters 3 and 9). In reflective writing, however, the approach is iterative and insightful. As the paragraphs and sections unfold, the reader gains a sense of your reasoning as it changes and grows. Figure 10.1 illustrates what I mean by this, using a flow chart and some of Gina's work on holistic practice.

Activity 10.4   Critical thinking

Look back now at my insights revealed in the above passage about body image rehabilitation and then at the summary of Gina's shift in thinking shared in Figure 10.1. How do these revealed shifts in thinking make you feel? Did learning seem an accumulation of insights or a remoulding of what you think?

As this answer is based on your own observation, there is no outline answer at the end of the chapter.

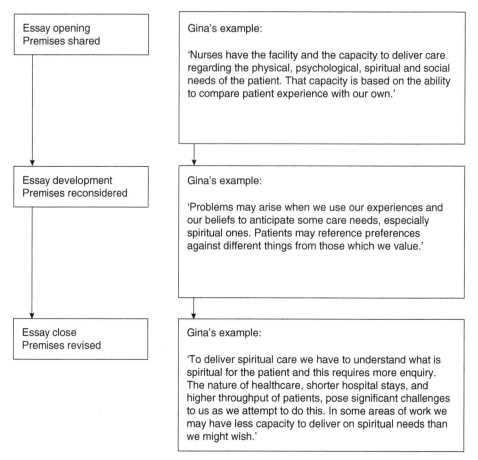

Figure 10.1 Reflecting and learning

Using reflective frameworks

Many students learn the process of reflective writing using one or another of the reflective practice frameworks (Kelsey and Hayes, 2015). We 'frame' experiences in different ways and are then able (with colleagues) to discuss the perspectives that we develop, adopt or abandon along the way. Among the reflective frameworks commonly used within nursing courses are those proposed by Gibbs (1988). The Gibbs framework encourages us to:

1. *Clearly describe the situation.* Without premature judgement, state what happened or what we understand to be factual.

2. *Explore our feelings.* Feelings are often a filter through which we read events. Does this experience represent a threat, an accolade, a challenge or affirmation of what we do? Do feelings help me to understand what was happening?

3. *Evaluate the experience.* Was this positive, negative, confusing or ambiguous?

4. *Reflect.* Make sense of the experience. Do we have a chance to learn here and to confirm what counts as excellent or poor? Is this something that helps me to understand a wider range of healthcare issues?

5. *Conclude.* What do we take away from this? Can these lessons be applied elsewhere?

6. *Act.* What might we do differently in the future?

The very popular framework by Rolfe et al. (2011) asks the nurse to address questions in three distinct areas: *what?* (events and experiences), *so what?* (significance and consequences) and *what next?* (necessary actions or responses).

*   *What?* For example: What was happening? What were my feelings, and those that I surmise others had?
*   *So what?* For example: What is the significance of these events? What have been or could be the consequences of this?
*   *What next?* For example: What remains to be done? What is now mandated?

At their best, reflective frameworks help us to showcase our learning. As we consider matters such as the aesthetics of care, review the ways in which beliefs and feelings shaped what we did, we demonstrate both insight and change. At the end of the essay, we can state what we might do differently in the future because we can articulate what experience has taught us in the past. Writing using the reflective frameworks, however, requires a little thought. I recommend the following:

*   Start by making a series of points that you wish to write about and decide under which framework heading these will appear (otherwise, you might make the same point in more than one place).
*   If you find that there are no points for some framework headings, decide whether this matters.
*   Decide whether you wish to write about something rather bigger than the incident or care episode, perhaps relating to narratives and discourses you see developing over time with this patient (see Chapter 11).

Whether you are an advocate of a particular reflective framework depends upon your teaching to date and perhaps too on your level of confidence writing in a reflective manner. In my experience, more confident students find some frameworks restrictive. They observe that they have to shoehorn reflection into the framework. My advice is to work with your tutor. There is value in working with a particular framework as you build your confidence and then later to experiment with a looser form of reflective writing, perhaps when a course grade is not at issue.

Levels of reflective reasoning

During the 1980s, Honey and Mumford (1982) developed their typology of learning styles, arguing that different students had different aptitudes for particular sorts of learning. No single person was a pure-type learner, they argued, but we all have propensities to learn in particular ways. To learn in another style required additional effort. The four learning styles described by Honey and Mumford were *activists* (those who liked to learn through projects, practical enquiries or research), *theorists* (those who liked to build and relate new experience to existing theories), *reflectors* (those who liked to examine situations from the point of view of experience and different perspectives used there) and *pragmatists* (those who liked to solve problems, to produce outcomes that were tangible and confidence-boosting). Understanding learning styles is important because it may help to explain why writing at more sophisticated reflective reasoning levels can prove so difficult. You might be excellent at writing analytical essays (theorists often excel there) but find it much harder to develop a reflective approach to experience.

It can seem hard for students with other learning styles to 'reflect for reflection's sake', but in my experience it is possible to make headway when you give further and more familiar purpose to reflection. So, the theorist might use a series of reflections to build a theory that explains particular sorts of behaviour (e.g. aggression). The activist might develop reflections that are then tested out in practice enquiry (e.g. different ways to provide reassurance). The pragmatist might be encouraged to see reflection as one of the tools in the armoury of clarifying what constitutes a healthcare problem. Importantly, that work starts at the outset with the question, 'Does a problem exist in the first place?'

You will need to distinguish between levels of reflection to decide whether the essay you are preparing is operating at the required level.

Absolute reflection (lowest-level reflection)

In absolute reasoning, there is little or no introspection, little or no attention given to different interpretations of events. Instead, there is one absolute and personally reassuring perspective on care. Sometimes this is described as 'common sense'. Other competing perspectives, other possibilities, are dismissed as misguided at best. Descriptions of events are described with great conviction. You are sure the perspective you have adopted is the right one. You admit no doubt into your deliberations.

When I have encountered this way of thinking in students, I have explored with them some of the possible beliefs and values that underpin this viewpoint. Why does it seem hard to consider alternative perspectives, to admit to doubt within nursing practice? Here are two responses that I have received:

- Reflection is ineffective; it cannot bring about change, so why waste time and effort.
- People will always have different opinions. We cannot change those, so it is better to work on what can be proven and required.

Beliefs and values are powerful and frequently closely associated with our personal identity (Pickles et al., 2019). In healthcare, though, both of these responses are questionable.

If reflection were ineffectual, practitioners would not engage in risk analysis, understanding what arose in a near-miss situation. We know that dynamic healthcare relies upon our ability to reflect and then to act on reflections. It is certainly true that people hold a wide variety of opinions, and sometimes these are powerfully expressed. Nevertheless, refinements in care or policy are possible as opinions are reviewed, and better ways forward sought. For example, in 2021, the healthcare world is countering the Covid-19 pandemic. Different governments and agencies, such as the World Health Organization, are reviewing and updating expert opinion on how to tackle the threats posed by this virus (Smith and Judd, 2020). It is likely that mistakes will be made en route; but it seems clear that without the conviction that a best response can be agreed and built upon, little improvement would ensue.

Transitional reflection (low-level reflection)

Transitional reflection might be thought of as a cataloguing exercise, one in which you admit that there are many points to consider, many perspectives to understand, but that you will reveal comparatively little as regards your deductions. To refer to Rolfe et al.'s (2011) model, you are content to ask *what?* but are rather more circumspect about confiding your deductions in *so what?* At this level of reflection, you are less confident to draw conclusions about what a collection of observations and experiences add up to. You may believe that others have better reasoning than you, that this comes only with experience, as nurses accumulate a large number of care episodes to draw upon.

In transitional reflection, you acknowledge a range of possibilities. You understand that care can be read in different ways. You know, for example, that pain and pain relief are intertwined experiences. The experience of pain may be mediated by the patient's expectations of pain relief. Will pain be removed altogether or simply reduced? Meaning is constructed from experience, a process applying as much to nurses as to patients.

What is important in moving up and out of this level of reflective reasoning is a willingness to speculate. A number of deductions may follow from a series of observations in practice. None (at this stage) is proven or tested, none is absolute or reputation-defining. Instead, they are possibilities – notions about 'what this might all mean'. Sharing your speculations alerts the reader to the range of possibilities you have considered. They assure the reader that you have not prematurely concluded what is happening, but that you understand the need to reach some 'try it and see' explanations which you could test in practice.

Contextual reflection (higher-level reflection)

Students sometimes indicate that they think of context only in clinical or patient terms. Thinking is contextualised to a clinical field, a nursing role or an identified patient need. Contextual reflection, however, admits a wider range of contexts. It is the recognition of this which helps a marker to determine that you have reflected more successfully. Here are some possible contexts:

- *Your professional concerns and doubts.* Imagine you have explained at the start of your essay that you have been concerned to understand how you listen, how you attend to everything the patient says. You then reflect on your difficulty about asking patients to clarify their worries.
- *The nature of a problem.* As suggested above, problems are defined by people; they exist when people define something as problematic. If you focus your reflections in ways that attend very closely to how the problem is being defined by you and others, you are reflecting contextually.
- *A change under way.* There may be a shift in care or in ideas about best practice. The working relationship between the nurse and the patient may be changing. You are thinking contextually if you ponder experiences with close regard to that change, what characterises it and what it might mean for your work as a nurse.

Activity 10.5   Reflection

Before reading on, pause now to consider whether you think you have thought about context in clear enough terms in your past reflective writing. Had you thought of context as purely to do with the patient and their needs?

As this answer is based on your own observation, there is no outline answer at the end of the chapter.

Independent reflection (highest-level reflection)

Independent reflection is characterised by an ability to treat your own beliefs and values as one influence in care, but not one with more power than others. You concede that the world of healthcare is a place of competing values and attitudes, and that it is necessary to interrogate your own and others' attitudes to better determine how best to proceed. Independent reflection is, in this sense, truly philosophical; it explores issues relating to ethics, priorities, identity and meaning as care is negotiated.

I discussed this definition with Raymet, and here is how she phrased it:

> You are reflecting independently when you're not afraid to treat yourself as a player on the stage. It is like you are an actor and you're ready to examine the play and your part in it. So, you have stepped outside your role and you have asked, 'How is the way that I am thinking working with others?' If I sense that I don't understand something, I have to begin again and explore what might be meant.

Do you agree that the theatre analogy is brilliant? Independent reflection is brave; you are willing to scrutinise your values, beliefs and attitudes to see if they fit with those of others. You are willing to pause and ask difficult questions about whether you are being as therapeutic as you first thought. On the page, such writing has a startling effect. You are seeing care afresh. You dare to ask the questions that others have set aside. The reader is convinced that you have the insights to change practice; and while that might require the persuasion of others, you can explain what you have witnessed in a new light.

We can now summarise levels of reflective reasoning. At one extreme, there is little or no reflection present; you admit no other possibilities, explanations or perspectives to your own (absolute reasoning). In transitional reasoning, other possibilities and perspectives are admitted into the debate, but these are kept at arm's length. You resist deciding what these add up to. In contextual reflective reasoning, you not only share deductions, but you connect these to the chosen context of the reflection. The reflection is much better focused and purposeful. In independent reflective reasoning, a refreshing – sometimes even a startling – new insight is shared on the subject area. You think in a way that reveals the bigger picture of a situation and can treat your own part in it in an inquisitive, evaluative and critical way. This is the most creative, the most searching, and the highest level of reflective reasoning.

Chapter summary

Reflective writing requires just as much discipline as other forms of academic work because it attends to the interpretation of events and the representation of your learning, conclusions and planned next actions. You demonstrate to the reader the sense you have made of experience. Reflective writing will be clearer if you explain the purpose of a given essay, if you use reflective frameworks consistently and transparently, and if you arrange your points under the relevant section headings of the work. Remember to be clear what you are writing about – facts, perceptions, perspectives, narratives and discourses. You may feel that you have a natural aptitude for reflection and writing about experience. Alternatively, you may feel happier writing in other ways. Reflective writing, though, is an important discipline for nurses. Much of nursing care involves deliberating on messy issues, those relating to what the patient needs or might value. Much as we might wish best practice to be readily defined and supported by research evidence, this is often not the case. Nurses will continue deliberating on how best to proceed, and reflections upon experience remain important here.

Activities: brief outline answers

Activity 10.3 Critical thinking (page 161)

An economic conundrum lies at the heart of much nursing care: many demands are made upon care resources and there is a finite supply of nursing care (the nurse's time, skills and material resources). For that reason, difficult choices have to be made. Nurses have to manage client expectations, and this within the context of a welfare state system. Were the patient paying for care directly, then the contractual relationship might differ, the parties referring to their terms of agreement. In service, nurses might have to explain such competing demands and how clinical need is assessed.

Nursing care is ideally designed to be person-centred, the patient collaborating with the nurse on care decisions. But this is not the only ethos of nursing. Nurses hope to alleviate pain, and indeed in some circumstances may explain that to tolerate pain is counterproductive for recovery and rehabilitation. So, this is an ethical conundrum, whether to respect the rights of the patient or to press a cause that the nurse sees as beneficial to the patient's well-being. At issue is a question of expertise. The patient is the authority on preferred ways of coping, but the nurse may know more about the consequences of poorly controlled pain.

As you reflect on service, it is usually important to acknowledge the complexity of care decisions and approaches. It is relatively rare that one perspective is obviously correct.

Further reading

Bolton, G. and Delderfield, R. (2018) *Reflective Practice: Writing and Professional Development,* 5th edition. London: SAGE.

Reflective practice and writing are not limited to healthcare, so dipping into this book, which deals with the process more generally, is very valuable. The explanations of perspective and narrative are especially good.

Esterhuizen, P. (2019) *Reflective Practice in Nursing,* 4th edition. London: SAGE/Learning Matters.

This is a good source of information on reflective practice models and the process of reflecting in a methodical way. The text is accessible, practical and reassuringly 'how to'.

Useful website

www.patientstories.org.uk

This URL takes you to a collection of short films of patient stories that I think are a useful resource to help you practise your reflective skills. The obvious reflections here relate to patient experience of injury, illness or difficulty, and that prompts you to consider how healthcare service professionals might best respond. But it is also worth considering some of the bigger discourses that might surround the stories that patients tell us. For example, are patients partners when it comes to care? How active or passive do we expect them to be? There are important discourses surrounding patient care partnership. Another discourse that you might consider is consumerism. If patients are consumers of care, can they also be a partner in that care? This is an important debate as nurses review quality of service and expectations of healthcare services change. Discuss one or more of the short films to revisit what you understand by the terms 'narrative' and 'discourse'.

Chapter 11　Writing the clinical case study

Chapter aims

After reading this chapter, you will be able to:

- explain what a clinical case is, something that captures a patient in a care context;
- summarise what is important when choosing a clinical case to write about;
- set the scene for the clinical case study, capturing the reader's interest in what you have to share;
- explain why the case needs to be explained in a measured and dispassionate way before moving on to analysis;
- outline the role of evidence in the clinical case study;
- characterise the analytical writing needed as you discuss case insights and concerns;
- outline what is required when you write up your conclusions to the clinical case study.

Introduction

In Chapter 6, I highlighted the advantage of following one or more clinical case studies during practice placements on your course. Sometimes the narrative of care that we need to understand extends beyond the single reflective interlude. Sometimes understanding the patient, the evolving care relationship, is more important than understanding the event, especially if you work towards more person-centred care

(Price, 2019b). Now we come to the writing up of those case studies and some points about the value of the same with regard to critical thinking.

Clinical case studies have remained a recurring feature of medical practice writing, where they have a very clear purpose (see the further reading section at the end of the chapter). The clinical case study is used to spotlight some unusual feature of an illness or its management that the author believes will be of professional interest to colleagues (Sasaki et al., 2019). The purpose of the clinical case study (sometimes called a report) is to use practice experience to better inform the practice of others. A clinical case study in the medical sense is noteworthy not necessarily because the treatment was successful. Rather, it exists to shed light on what experience, as well as the use of related evidence, can teach us. In the context of this book, clinical case studies have a very useful function, which is to illuminate template thinking, the way in which one practitioner (or team) tackled a particular need or problem. Nurses relate to patients as people, negotiating care through perceived needs. That which the patient achieves during care is as much to do with how patients feel and relate to healthcare staff as the efficacy of particular treatment. The nurse negotiates rather than prescribes care. In this, the nursing clinical case study is unique; it centres upon the patient and their context as much as upon an illness and any treatment.

In the past, 'nursing care studies' were written by students, often to illustrate a model of nursing in action. One of the problems of such studies, however, was that they could become unduly descriptive. It was relatively easy to write a simple account of care when what was really required was an illustration of critical thinking. For case study writing to work well, there needs to be a problem analysed, a conundrum explained, an insight gained and reviewed, something that sets the case in context and enables the nurse to demonstrate what is now understood about delivering patient care over a period of time.

Today, a clinical case study can (Price, 2017):

- explore the nature of person-centred care;
- illustrate how experience contributes to best practice;
- examine the linkage of evidence and practice (e.g. the case study might illustrate gaps in evidence or indicate where evidence of different sorts might usefully be combined);
- demonstrate higher-level critical thinking and reflection in action (case studies are an excellent way to explore the templates that nurses use to reason care).

Activity 11.1   Critical thinking

What do you think a clinical case study offers that a theory essay or a reflective episode account cannot?

Jot down your answers before turning to the outline answer at the end of the chapter.

Selecting the case

I have already indicated some of the key features of a patient's circumstances that might make them a good case to explore as part of your practice placement learning (see Chapter 6). All of those still hold good, but the selection of which case study to write up for assessment, or perhaps a paper for publication, requires some further thought. Most obviously, the patient's case has to fit with the objectives of a module of study (or else the requirements of a journal). If the module of study is on mental health, then clearly that must feature strongly within the case that you write up. Beyond that, though, there should be something about the case that allows you to demonstrate how you are interrogating experience, exploring the concepts in use and evaluating necessary skills. It is not enough that the patient evoked compassion, that they were articulate or friendly. Study of the patient's circumstances and nursing response has to exhibit how you and other nurses thought differently.

Case study: Elijah 1

To explain the planning and writing work with a case study, I am going to share a story about Elijah. Picture a 71-year-old man who suffered from Covid-19 pneumonia, necessitating a two-week stay in an intensive care unit (ICU). Elijah was extremely ill, nursed on a ventilator; and after being weaned off that, he was cared for within a rehabilitation unit, which forms the location for the case study.

In some regards, Elijah had much in common with other Covid-19 victims. The illness exhausted him and it took a long time for him to improve his lung function afterwards. What was important, however, were some rapidly developing delusions that followed his intensive care experience, in a patient without a history of prior mental illness. Elijah suffered a number of delusions about what had been done to him in the ICU. This centred upon a physiotherapist who was trying to help him recover now. Elijah's rehabilitation was affected by the delirium that followed his time on a ventilator.

Elijah's case above highlights the importance of finding the right focus for analysis. He has been chosen because his case highlights some problems met during rehabilitation. While there is an established history of delirium associated with ventilator treatment, Elijah's context is more interesting still. He suffered an illness that people from black and ethnic minority populations have proved especially vulnerable to; and in a module that explores mental health, the case is well chosen. In traditional teaching about the consequences of artificial ventilation, what represents appropriate care might not apply for a patient such as Elijah. In his case, the delirium did not present as a general agitation, sometimes described as 'hyperactive delirium' (Hyde-Wyatt, 2014); it focused progressively on a series of delusions and finally upon an aggressive outburst.

Experience has a teaching role to play. Delirium (confusion, agitation, or conversely withdrawal) is a widespread experience after ICU care, but Elijah's presentation of it was atypical and it posed questions about arranging person-centred care.

Writing the context introduction

University requirements for the setting out of clinical case studies may vary, but I would recommend an introduction that sets the context of the case study. The role of the introduction is to bring to the reader's attention why this case study is noteworthy. What about the patient or their care marks the work as remarkable in some regard? Classically, case studies are introduced for the following reasons:

- they highlight a previously poorly articulated or unmet problem that deserves analysis;
- they exemplify a feature of care negotiation, perhaps that which illuminates care philosophy or a key skill;
- they highlight something important about the interface between evidence and practice, or perhaps between theory and that which is realisable in care;
- they articulate the resolution of dilemmas (the case study of Elijah might equally have centred on whether it was ethical to treat his delirium with an antipsychotic medication).

While clinical case study writing should be measured and analytical, this does not mean that it should be introduced drily. The introduction should interest the reader. The case study may be an assignment answer, but it should have professional merit too – it should seem valuable to another nurse.

In the example of Elijah, several contexts seem important. The first concerns delirium and recovery after time spent on a ventilator. Delirium takes different forms; it may be hyperactive (classically, the patient is agitated and anxious), intermediate or hypoactive (the patient is withdrawn and difficult to engage with) (Hayhurst et al., 2016). But to varying degrees too, the patient might experience hallucinations and delusions about what happened in the ICU or what is happening now. The question arises: How shall we best counter delirium?

The second context relates to care philosophy. Like other Covid-19 victims, Elijah faced an acute admission to hospital that quickly deteriorated into an emergency situation where he required mechanical ventilation. There was scant time for nurses to build a rapport with Elijah, to negotiate care in an adequately person-centred way. Care negotiation had to play catch-up after a frightening experience. The question arises: How do you make care person-centred in these circumstances?

The third context was associated with Elijah's background. As a man of colour, as well as being at risk from Covid-19 because of his age and gender, Elijah faced considerable uncertainty. It was important, then, to support him in a sensitive way, reassuring him as much as possible. He experienced ICU care as a racially linked threat. Helping Elijah had to involve understanding his perceptions of events and appreciating the cultural sensitivities that this might involve.

Here is an extract paragraph from the introduction to the case study where I try to capture the reader's professional interest in this case.

Case study: Elijah 2

Nurses hope to partner patients in care, to negotiate care measures from a position of mutual respect. Sometimes, however, person-centred care relationships must start from another place, one where it is exceptionally hard to empower patients. Sometimes the care negotiations begin where the patient feels disempowered, suspicious, and where the nurse must use all of their skills to help the patient feel secure. Whatever best practice guidelines we have for person-centred care, they presume a collabora-tive starting point. When a 71-year-old patient, Elijah (name adjusted), is admitted to hospital acutely ill with Covid-19-related pneumonia, however, where they are rapidly transferred to the ICU and artificial ventilation, the care negotiating begins post-traumatic event. Care is negotiated against a significant power imbalance where the patient is severely disadvantaged. It is then heightened further when efforts to build rapport with the patient during rehabilitation are complicated by delirium, the patient rapidly developing a series of delusions about his ICU care and the motives of a therapist who is trying to assist him with his breathing and mobility exercises now.

Activity 11.2   Critical thinking

Compare the above opening paragraph on the clinical case study of Elijah against the classical reasons for writing a case study (bullet points above). Which of those seems likely to be addressed in this start to the case study? How do I secure the reader's interest in this case study?

An outline answer is given at the end of the chapter.

Writing the case description

One of the things that marks out your case study writing as analytical is the disciplined way in which sections are set out. If the opening of the paper has been to set a scene and capture the reader's interest, the next section exists to describe the case as directly, cleanly and accurately as possible. The case in our instance describes a man and his rehabilitation care, now complicated by delirium. This is the most descriptive part of the paper that you write, although you will need to plan it in a very analytical way. A good way to describe this section is to see it as akin to the way in which a police officer might describe a crime scene. It is important to present all of the relevant facts, those relating to the time and place of the sequence of events. Importantly, though, the police officer does not interpret the scene at this stage; there are no speculative points about needs, motives, relationships or values. The case description describes that which happened, as factually as possible.

I asked Sue (our case study registered nurse) about how that might seem in order to better illustrate what is required. Here is what she said:

> *I think nurses habitually start to interpret experiences and to infer needs and wishes. We want to comfort people. We have become relatively good at second-guessing what is required in different situations. That's not what you want in a case study, though, is it? You should stand back first, describe something, and only then explain your insights afterwards. You don't want to muddy the water, making it harder for the reader to understand how your response fitted with what happened.*

Sue has expressed the key requirement brilliantly. If the reader is to make sense of what the case teaches, then a clear separation has to be made between events and reasoning. We have to set aside our urgent need to interpret and to solve problems. No matter how intuitively we might approach care, there is a need to explain reasoning to others, which requires us to describe a case cleanly in the first instance.

So, in the case study of Elijah, we need a brief account of the chronological events that took place. We need an account of what the patient said or did so that we can appreciate it starkly. We must resist the temptation to interpret it prematurely: 'Of course, Elijah was anxious because …' We have to decide what slice of time the case study focuses upon. It might be possible to outline the whole of Elijah's time in hospital. Many clinical case studies centre upon a section of time, that which best exemplifies what is of interest in the case study.

Here are three paragraphs of writing about the case that exemplify this very factual focus, this dispassionate report of events and words. They might seem cold to you if you have been used to other reflective forms of writing, but they lend to the case study an objective starting point.

Case study: Elijah 3

Elijah spent a total of seven weeks in hospital, first two days on an assessment ward, where despite oxygen therapy his condition deteriorated rapidly, then two weeks on the ICU where he was sedated on an artificial ventilator. After being weaned off the

(Continued)

(Continued)

ventilator, he was transferred to a rehabilitation ward where he spent the remaining time (the subject period for this case study). During this rehabilitation period, the patient continued to receive supplemental oxygen using nasal cannula, and he began a programme of physiotherapy to counter his residual dyspnoea, reduce the risks associated with immobility, and begin building his confidence again after what he described as a terrifying event. The physiotherapy regimen consisted of two daily sessions superintended by a therapist, supplemented by two lighter breathing exercise sessions led by the nurse.

During the course of his rehabilitation sessions, Elijah became incrementally more suspicious and then aggressive when the physiotherapist worked with him. The nurses asked him whether he was fearful of what exercising his lungs might do after such an acute illness. They explained that the exercise regime was carefully calibrated to work within his personal limits. On the third day of his rehabilitation exercise regime, Elijah lashed out at the physiotherapist and her assistant, knocking her to the floor. He glared at her from his bed and bellowed, 'What are you doing to me! Who are you anyway? Do they pay you for this! Did they send you to finish the job?!' When the team reviewed this incident and his care leading up to it, they noted that Elijah had started to express severe doubts about the physiotherapist he had assaulted. He had started to rehearse memories that he felt he had from his time in the ICU.

The senior nurse interviewed Elijah and he insisted that he remembered the physiotherapist from before. She had hurt him when he was ill in the ICU (the therapist had no role there, it being a separate red zone isolation facility). Elijah claimed that she had pinched and bruised him. He believed that he had heard her laughing at him. 'They have such low pain thresholds and not an ounce of fight in them', he reported recalling what he believed the therapist had said. The senior nurse reminded Elijah that she had enquired about his ICU experience before, when he had first arrived on the rehabilitation ward. Then he had said that he had no particular memories, just of feeling ill, breathless and frightened. Now he insisted that the physiotherapist had pinched and humiliated him while in the ICU.

What I hope you note in this example is that the case unfolds the problem. In this instance, that centres on patient beliefs and behaviour. Elijah was not obviously agitated, but as time progressed post-ICU he became convinced that he had been persecuted there. The nurse also checked that there had been no derogatory remarks directed at Elijah in the ICU and that his sedation had been well managed. The nurse established that the physiotherapist had indeed not worked in the ICU. But at this point, no analysis is undertaken. There is no speculation about the effects of sedatives, hypoxia, his state of anxiety when he became ill and was transferred to intensive care. Later, a debate might follow about care standards and respect for the patient. Elijah's memory could be a delirium delusion or it could have a basis in truth. This section, though, is not a place to speculate about Elijah's perceptions of what happened. The purpose is to record what he believed occurred.

Before a problem can be solved, it must be described as clearly and dispassionately as possible. If the patient does not trust those caring for them, collaboration on care becomes difficult. With Elijah, the case description then went on to outline what the nurse then did to address his anxieties. This consisted of four things:

- She introduced the diary entries of the nurses who had cared for him in the ICU. This detailed their names and what they did for him, as well as the routine of his day. The diary entries also included a summary of how he was progressing there.
- She arranged for his lead ICU nurse to speak to him via video call on a mobile phone (Covid-19 protection measures precluded a personal visit from a red zone area). The nurse described how she had looked after him, moving him regularly, watching over him and controlling the machines that breathed for him.
- She described to him how a strange and technical environment, no obvious night or day, medications, and hypoxia can serve to disorientate a patient and evoke vivid memories. Patients might suffer hallucinations or delusions.
- She reviewed Elijah's skin with him in order to ascertain whether there were any marks indicative of recent pinching or other forms of injury. No marks were identified.

The case description detailed that no further physical attacks upon staff followed, but Elijah remained convinced that the same therapist had malevolent intent towards him. The team then elected to assign to Elijah's care a different therapist and continued with their psychological work, piecing together with him the narrative of his illness and care. As no further aggressive outburst followed, he did not receive antipsychotic medication. Elijah eventually left the rehabilitation ward with improved respiratory function and an improving level of mobility, but entrenched beliefs that the particular therapist had been a threat.

Activity 11.3   Reflection

Why should the case description of your paper be presented very factually, without undue interpretation? What might be problematic if you used it to speculate prematurely?

An outline answer is given at the end of the chapter.

Summarising relevant evidence

So far, the clinical case study has set the scene, creating a focus for the paper, and it has dispassionately described the case. The case has been a patient and his care over a period of time on the rehabilitation ward. We now need to utilise any available evidence that played – or could have played – a role in the case. Not every clinical case study will have a large body of evidence to summarise. Sometimes evidence is sparse, or even non-existent in some areas. But the point of this section is to succinctly summarise evidence that you believe has a bearing on the case in question. The evidence might indicate support for the care measures used or it might raise questions about the care approach. It might be contradictory, with some evidence countering other evidence. The point is that this section sets a wider world of knowledge context to the case in question.

As you have read earlier in Chapter 8, evidence can take different forms, and all of it might be relevant to your chosen clinical case study. You will have to discriminate, though, between what has real purchase for the issue or problem in question and what is much more peripheral and can reasonably be left out. The purpose of this section is not to provide a thorough literature review. It is not an evidence review paper, but an evidence in possible application summary. For that reason, the range of evidence that you might include here may well be rather more circumscribed. It is evidence that has a good fit with the context, with the need or problem identified.

Activity 11.4 Speculation

What evidence do you think might have purchase in a case study such as that of Elijah?

Jot down your answer before reading on.

I hope that you immediately suggested evidence relating to delirium, which causes confusion and anxiety for a patient in or after intensive care. You might have ventured that you would look at evidence relating to beliefs and values, how they are formed and sustained in the context of illness and beyond. Elijah believed that he was being persecuted; irrespective of whether that was factually true, his response to those helping him was sincerely based on the beliefs held. Other evidence of interest includes remedial measures designed to counter delirium in the context of intensive care and its immediate aftermath. Delirium can be tackled using antipsychotic medication (e.g. haloperidol) but it might also be addressed using occupational health or psychological measures (Cavallazzi et al., 2012).

It seems unlikely that Elijah was maltreated within the ICU. The claimed perpetrator did not work there, and a survey of the skin revealed no marks or injuries. Elijah was one of several very sick patients in care at the same time and the ICU staff sought to rescue each. However, because we cannot dismiss abuse out of hand, it would be relevant to review any evidence relating to the mistreatment of sedated patients within high-dependency care areas. It would be especially relevant to examine any evidence relating to memory of that heard while under different levels of sedation. While nurses might not like to confront the possibility of maltreatment in care, we should not be complacent.

In this section, you review the nature and extent of the evidence available, whether it seems to relate to the clinical case study in question. Once again, the writing style should be objective and measured. It is not appropriate to jump to conclusions and judge the match of clinical case study care and evidence. Insights and issues are discussed in the next section, so here you are still laying a reasoning trail for the reader, helping them to take stock of what you are considering. Take a look now at some further sample writing from this section of the case study. Here, I am taking stock of the adequacy of evidence available. Is the body of evidence clear and unambiguous? I have not yet applied it to Elijah; I am still reviewing all that might be relevant.

Case study: Elijah 4

The above selection of reviewed papers highlights a series of difficulties regarding evidence-based practice and the management of post-ICU delirium. The first is that clinicians vary in their assessment of the significance of delirium. Some 80 per cent of post-ICU patients may suffer a degree of delirium (Weaver et al., 2017), but for the majority it is transitory and relatively easily combatted with reassurance by clinicians. When authors determine that the problem is significant, however, distinctions are made between hypoactive delirium (withdrawal and disengagement) and hyperactive delirium (characterised by anxiety, agitation, and sometimes delusions and hallucinations). The literature varies in its assessment as to which is more important. Hypoactive delirium may undermine rehabilitation as the patient gives up hope, while hyperactive delirium risks self-harm (e.g. the patient ripping out tubes).

Beyond debates regarding the nature of the problem, division then arises as regards best response. Weaver et al. (2017) researched the merits of antipsychotic drugs in terms of the speed with which patients recovered from delirium. They deduced that there was no obvious merit in the use of medications such as haloperidol, which could risk cardiac function in patients that may have been ventilated artificially. Patient counselling or coaching solutions offered a similarly incomplete answer as patients varied in their levels of agitation, as well as how counselling support was then used. There was, however, modest indication that explaining ICU care to patients (continuity follow-up) might benefit patients as they narrated what had happened to them (Haines et al., 2019).

Activity 11.5   Reflection

A question arises as you move towards the next section of your case study, and this centres on the fit of evidence to the circumstances described. In Chapter 8, I described how different types of research might be evaluated.

In the clinical case study, however, the focus is on how evidence relates to experience, and vice versa. Each of the following questions might assist you as you weigh up what evidence has to offer:

1. How coherent is the body of evidence? If research recommends many different and divergent things, the utility value of evidence might currently be low.

2. Conversely, does the body of evidence suggest that some patient experiences or needs are more important and/or occur more frequently?

3. Does the evidence suggest that one or more interventions are more effective, or else better understood, better received or better evaluated by patients?

4. Does the evidence suggest that something remains ambiguous or contentious? It is here that difficulties might arise for the patient and clinician.

5. Are there any evidence 'black holes' where no one has apparently confronted issues that arose in the case study? Your case study might point to the need for future research.

Think back to a patient that you have nursed in order to judge whether the above evidence in use questions seem valuable. Does this help you to clarify in your mind why sometimes the relevance of evidence is at least as important as its apparent power (e.g. sample size, robust fieldwork methods)?

As this is a personal reflection, no outline answer is offered at the end of the chapter.

Discussing insights and issues

In the penultimate section of your case study, you bring together all of the important points, discussing insights and issues about what the case might teach us. This includes that which was observed from practice and that which is available elsewhere from evidence. It enables you to review what seemed wise, practicable and desirable to the clinician in practice. It considers how the clinicians proceeded, the decisions that they made. In some instances, the nurse might have been unaware of valuable evidence – their practice template was perhaps incomplete. But in other instances, the reasoning may have accommodated factors that research and theorists failed to consider. Sharing insights and issues demonstrates to the reader what you thought significant about the case study and the wider evidence available.

This is often the longest section of the clinical case study, but it still needs to be a disciplined form of writing that shows how you drill down to what is really important. To that end, it is useful to identify and note down the four or perhaps five most important points before you write up the section. My maxim is that it is better to write about fewer things more clearly than it is to range widely, explaining matters ambiguously.

Let us return to the Elijah case study. Here are some points that I speculated as important from the case study:

1. Delirium is not simply a product of altered physiology, medications and treatments. Delirium is experienced individually, and in this case Elijah experiences the insecurities of illness/ICU in racial persecution terms. While there was no objective evidence of mistreatment and the physiotherapist had no contact with the patient in the ICU, Elijah's future care relationship is impacted by his fears and beliefs. It remains debatable whether clinicians can in a short space of time counter deeply held beliefs that may have been informed by past personal experiences. Asking another therapist to work with Elijah was a practical interim step, however.

2. There is a debate about inoculating patients against delirium. The senior nurse used three explanatory measures as a rescue for Elijah, but what if these had been used more strategically to tell his story in the ICU before? This raises questions about how serious delirium is, whether it warrants preventative work.

3. What does Elijah's case tell us about delivering person-centred care in a post-psychological trauma context? Person-centred care starts with the patient's own narrative of need and concern. This case seems to accent that attention needs to focus firmly on Elijah's perceived concerns and needs if he is to partner the nurse in care.

4. Do we really recognise delirium in all of its presentations? Hypoactive delirium (non engagement, a withdrawn patient rather than agitation, delusions or hallucinations) may in the longer term hamper rehabilitation even more if the patient gives up hope of recovery. Are our patient assessment working templates complete?

5. Might other factors have contributed to Elijah's perceptions, fears and aggressive behaviour? For example, there is no mention of him having any contact with family or friends during hospitalisation. Perhaps if there had been, he might have felt less vulnerable. Even where social contact might be possible, it is constrained by Covid-19 protocols, such as wearing personal protective equipment (PPE), which presents a barrier to communication. Could this have exacerbated Elijah's anxieties and fears?

Here is an example of my musing:

Case study: Elijah 5

In the midst of a pandemic, care resources are stretched to the limit. As patients emerge from ICUs, there is a considerable degree of relief, but recognition too that residual work remains to be done. In the case of Elijah, this certainly centred on physical rehabilitation. There was a clearly reasoned regimen of breathing exercises and graduated mobility training to help Elijah recover his independence. But what also seems certain is that mental health rehabilitation is important as well. Person-centred care (Price, 2019b) highlights how the nurse tries to discover the patient's own narrative of injury or illness, their coping and recovery. That seems important in the case of a patient with confusing, frightening and alarming thoughts about what has been happening to them. If the memories are inaccurate, then they still need to be understood. The patient still needs assistance to make sense of their experiences and beliefs so that next step care can be contemplated together. Elijah was not simply another Covid-19 sufferer, an ICU survivor; he was a patient trying to make sense of a gap in his recent history, but who still needed physiotherapy now.

Activity 11.6 Reflection

Think back to some other essays that you have written and consider the following maxim also given at the start of this section:

> *Writing about less, but in rather more detail, is better than writing about a lot superficially.*

Do you support the maxim? If you have tried to stretch too far, writing widely before, was that because you imagined that an assessor wanted to know what you knew rather than how you reasoned? If you focused your work more, what gave you the confidence to do that?

As this is a personal reflection, no outline answer is offered at the end of the chapter.

Reaching conclusions

The final section (as in other essays) is made up of your conclusions. You finish the clinical case study by summing up what you deduce from the enquiry. As with other conclusions, it is important to focus this one on what was discussed in the preceding sections of the paper – you should not be raising new issues at this point. The conclusions should relate closely to what you have speculated about in the last section, as well as to the marrying of evidence and experience. You might wonder what constitutes a conclusion, the point where speculation ends. The answer is that a conclusion is where you state your resting position, where you let go of the discussion. Experienced nurses rarely write diatribes in their conclusion. The deductions are measured and nuanced, as befits higher-level critical thinking (see Chapter 3).

Here is a sample paragraph from my conclusion to the Elijah clinical case study. Notice how closely it relates to the speculative points that I raised in the last section of the paper. It is something that I relate to person-centred care and rehabilitation, the introductory context that I started the clinical case study with. A good conclusion brings the reader full circle, back to that which first alerted them to the possible significance of the case study.

Case study: Elijah 6

The case study of Elijah offers a salutary lesson about care investment. What seems to mark out the expertise of the nurse is not simply what they say or do, but when they choose to do it. Expert person-centred care is about timely investment. In this instance, the senior nurse uses information to rescue the care of Elijah. She offers diary accounts of his ICU time, a personal greeting from a nurse caring for him there, and an explanation of delirium to help Elijah explain feelings of persecution to himself. She ventures the argument, 'We cannot always trust our memories for these reasons, but here is an account of what was done to help you – you were important to my colleagues.'

This can represent a patch to counter emergent problems. It can, though, when used earlier, represent an inoculation of care. The measures used help to personalise care and assure the patient of proper regard for their needs. What remains problematic, however, is judging when the patient is ready to engage in such a review of events. When Elijah transferred to the rehabilitation ward, he expressed no delusional thoughts. In such circumstances, even against significant time restraints, it might be wise to offer a 'just in case' account anyway. From such an account, new narratives of need and care might begin.

Chapter summary

Clinical case studies offer an excellent opportunity to analyse care over more protracted periods of time, to work with the more familiar care currency (working with a patient and their needs). This seems especially relevant in person-centred care.

The clinical case study can serve a number of different professional and academic purposes (e.g. unpicking a problem, relating evidence and experience to each other). Importantly, in this book, case studies can help us to explore how the nurse reasons, revealing the templates that they use to deliver care.

Writing up a clinical case study, though, requires a disciplined writing approach. The case must be chosen with care and with regard to module assessment requirements. Thereafter, the study has to be arranged in a series of strategic sections and utilise a measured, dispassionate form of writing. Each section of the clinical case study builds on the last, and it is important to avoid judging points until issues are discussed and conclusions are reached at the end.

Activities: brief outline answers

Activity 11.1 Critical thinking (page 170)

I would suggest that the clinical case study offers the chance to relate how care was negotiated and planned. This is rarely captured in a reflective practice essay, with its focus on a clinical episode. It is something much more applied than that typically discussed in a theory-based essay. Here, you are able to acknowledge how nurses think in practice, to discover what is sometimes called 'practice wisdom'. Practice is a place of learning, and the clinical case study exemplifies that.

Activity 11.2 Critical thinking (page 173)

I venture that this writing promises the analysis of a care problem and it examines care philosophy (person-centred care). I wonder if you felt that the writing attracts you because it raises the question of what happened next. How did they address this problem? In professional writing (for nursing journals), this is called the hook. It draws you into the discussion. A journal reader does not have to read to pass assessments, so the writing has to be professionally compelling.

Activity 11.3 Reflection (page 176)

If you move too quickly to analyse the case, speculating the significance of events, it is then much harder for the reader to distinguish between the events and your interpretations of need. You risk muddying the analysis; were you to do that, an examiner might wonder what you had left out. If you offer only interpretation and no situation, it is difficult to demonstrate your reasoning ability.

Further reading

It is interesting to examine how case studies are used in textbooks.

Cummings, L. (2016) *Case Studies in Communication Disorders.* Cambridge: Cambridge University Press.

This book, as others, cuts to the chase cataloguing classic communication problems and recommending ways to proceed in response. *In extremis*, the approach can feel like a formulaic solution to therapeutic work.

Farne, H., Norris-Cervetto, E. and Warbeck-Smith, J. (2015) *Oxford Cases in Medicine and Surgery*, 2nd edition. Oxford: Oxford University Press.

This book offers a reassuringly wide range of classic patient presentations that the clinician might be confronted with and details how to conduct an assessment. It is worth reflecting on to what extent a patient need is adequately defined by disease, illness or injury presentation. Nonetheless, it is a book that illustrates medical template reasoning in action.

Page, K. and McKinney, A. (eds) (2012) *Nursing the Acutely Ill Adult: Case Book*. Milton Keynes: Open University Press.

Karen Page and Aidín McKinney offer a hybrid approach to analysing clinical care requirements. In many ways, the textbook mimics the medical textbook approach, but there is also a clear recognition that patients interpret their own problems – and that can be either a resource or a challenge.

Price, B. (2019) *Delivering Person-Centred Care in Nursing*. London: SAGE/Learning Matters.

My own textbook offers an investigative approach to person-centred care with a clear emphasis on understanding what patients say (their narratives). In this book, the patient comes first, constituting the context for all subsequent discussion of problems and working solutions.

Useful websites

There is a wealth of video illustration of clinical case study presentation and analysis available online, especially on YouTube. If you wish to explore widely, then simply search for 'clinical case studies' there. I would like, though, to direct you to two sample YouTube video clips in order to make some points:

www.youtube.com/watch?v=mpE-oaix5kA

In this video, *Case Study Clinical Example: Session with a Client with Bipolar Disorder (Fluctuations in Mood)* by Judith Johnson, we meet Tom in conversation with his therapist, who is taking his history of problems while at university and beyond. This nicely illustrates how a case study can tell a story over time, as a series of episodes or stages. Sometimes clinicians need to understand that journey; it becomes a unit of care or therapy. Notice how the therapist regularly summarises Tom's account and invites him to interpret events for himself. The case study enables us to see how a clinician helps to shape the representation of patient experiences so that it is amenable to treatment. The clinician is using her template reasoning to help map Tom's concerns and needs.

www.youtube.com/watch?v=Mew2wzpuhTs

This video is entitled *How to Present a Patient Case: The Signpost Method*. In medical education, case study presentation is a routine way in which doctors learn to diagnose illness and recommend a treatment plan. But there seems no reason at all why this method cannot be adapted to clinical learning in nursing too. Case study presentation is an excellent way to explore person-centred care and expose template reasoning. See what you think.

Chapter 12 Building and using your portfolio of learning

Chapter aims

After reading this chapter, you will be able to:

- outline how by using a portfolio, you can build learning that crosses course module boundaries;
- describe why it is important to connect concepts to practice, exploring that which is workable as well as professional;
- use chosen themes to explore practice and possible improvements there;
- build or augment your learning log in ways that show how your thinking has changed over time, working towards successful template reasoning.

Introduction

We have reached the final chapter of this book and come full circle, back to where we started in Chapter 1, with its description of critical thinking and the recommendation that thinking has a professional purpose. We think critically not only to pass course assessments, but also to move towards the sort of imaginative and responsive template reasoning that nurses use in practice (Alfayoumi, 2019). What starts as a study of 'what' (e.g. the disease, the theory) becomes incrementally a study of why we practice as we do (e.g. ethical reasons) to end with a much greater appreciation of how care is successfully delivered by nurses (e.g. practice templates) (Jessee, 2018). An additional literature exists on clinical reasoning (see the recommendations at the end of the chapter), but you need to understand the journey to that. The learning narrative of your course is fundamentally one of both subject coverage (module topics) and skill development, that which entails critical thinking and reflection. Portfolio-building is part of that journey (Lai and Wu, 2016; Peddle et al., 2016).

The rationale of portfolios

All sorts of people develop portfolios, not least nurses. It is worth pausing for a moment to consider what such portfolios are meant to do. They are at once an exercise in development (compiling them helps you learn to strategise) and an outcome proof of achievement. An artist carries to meetings with patrons a collection of past works that have already been completed which they hope seem impressive. The portfolio in nursing works in a very similar way. Building the portfolio is a disciplined professional exercise, but it serves a proof of ability as well (Peddle et al., 2016). It is something that you can show to others, submit as part of course assessment, or incorporate as evidence for job applications. It is not simply something that you 'have to do as part of the course'.

One of the problems of any portfolio is that its contents can seem fragmentary. The fact that your course is arranged in a modular form helps to organise the subject matter of nursing but it potentially fragments the account of developing skills (Oermann et al., 2018). There is a risk that you learn a great deal about the 'what' and the 'why' of nursing, but then neglect the 'how' of nursing, the ways in which needs are answered by information. You need as many bridges as possible to help you to apply theory and research to practice, and then in turn to take lessons from practice back into theory-building. What portfolios need is some kind of narrative, which in nursing is closely associated with skills. If the artist sells a style or vision, the nurse sells a purposeful use of skills.

Concepts and templates

In Chapter 1, I introduced you to templates, the ways in which practised nurses sensitively, effectively and efficiently respond to care needs, working with patients and others to find the right ways forward. Such templates combine experience, reflections and insights, research evidence, and theory to help justify the courses of action adopted (Ray-Barruel et al., 2019). The templates span the theory–practice gap and suggest ways in which you have taken ideas from your learning and used them skilfully in your care. To do that, nurses have to conceptualise nursing activity in different ways. Here are some concepts that regularly recur in nursing practice (it is no coincidence that they are strongly skill-centred):

- patient teaching (teaching is a concept closely related to counselling and supporting, and may be used in concert with patients);
- comforting (reassurance is probably important, but therapeutic use of touch as well, perhaps companionable silence too);
- listening (active listening, in ways that attend closely to what the patient explains);
- planning (this is so often reduced to a discussion of care plans, but it is bigger than that – it is about strategy, coordination and liaison, with patients and others);
- problem-solving (includes problem identification, mapping, option analysis and collaboration).

The ability to think using concepts, to switch and adjust them, is what helps you to develop the sort of working templates that the most skilful nurses use in practice (Friberg, 2019). Templates connect clinical experience and your learning, building concepts to use as part of care that seems timely, apt and person-centred. For example, unless we know what we mean by active listening, problem-solving with a patient becomes that much harder. We have to adequately hear what concerns the patient and identify what – within experience, theory or research evidence – can then serve them well (Stojan et al., 2016).

I want to propose to you, then, that it is a very good idea to build within your portfolio a series of overarching concept-led records that incrementally shift focus from what you need to know to how you might use that in care. This is more than a log of things experienced or taught. Let me illustrate that with listening once more. Imagine that you make listening one of the recurring themes within your portfolio. There are different aspects of listening to attend to. In your earliest modules of study, attention might focus on the theory of listening, as part of communication. Listening, of course, operates in different contexts (e.g. the anxious patient, the dying patient), and that too affects how listening is done. Incrementally, though, it is possible to build in more and more reflections on the nuances of listening. These will be reflections on things such as the emotional effort of listening and on encounters where listening did or did not work so well. We will be shifting towards practice and towards templates for good practice. We will be shifting incrementally from 'what', through 'why' to 'how'. This becomes a narrative of skill development.

Activity 12.1   Reflection

You might be reading this book at almost any point in your studies, or indeed beyond as a registered nurse preparing work for revalidation (NMC, 2019). Regardless, answer the following questions before turning to my responses at the end of the chapter:

1. What do you think are the benefits of building a narrative through your portfolio, on chosen concepts that are central to nursing care?

2. Who might you discuss your plans with, ensuring that the concepts help to characterise your ability as a nurse?

3. What sorts of things can fuel your chosen concepts, that which you return to again in your entries within the portfolio?

An outline answer is given at the end of this chapter.

Choosing or designing a portfolio of your own

When portfolios were first developed in nurse education, they were usually in a paper form. Today, portfolios might be built and updated on your computer (Lai and Wu, 2016). In the beginning, portfolios were designed in printed sections, as forms to be filled out. Universities now vary in the extent to which your portfolio is in a set format. For example, it might be a learning log, or alternatively something that facilitates rather more explorative and expressive writing. As a registered nurse, you are not required to keep a portfolio in quite the same way. You will, however, need to amass a record of your continuing development, that relating to ongoing study, hours of completed practice, patient evaluations of your work, and reflections on practice (NMC, 2019). That record could become eclectic and poorly coordinated. It will not surprise you to learn, then, that I recommend you connect the different elements together using one or more themes of enquiry. There is no reason why your revalidation work cannot focus on a theme that you feel excited about.

The challenge in building a portfolio is how to combine the requirement for a record of study (I will call this the learning log) with something that demonstrates reasoning and reflective development. You will need both, a map (as it were) of where you have been, and a means of showing how you are thinking now and for the future. Here, then, I recommend that if your university portfolio is highly structured and closely related to the module of current study, you consider adding in some concept-led records which extend beyond the module and show your reasoning progression across the course. Perhaps these are added at the back of the record or in a complementary folder. These can take a very simple form (loose-leaf or paper record) that covers the following information:

1. *The selected conceptual theme and the date that was started.* This will become a section heading in your chosen record. Let us imagine that you have chosen listening as an essential concept or skill within nursing. Ideally, you have discussed your selections with your personal tutor, given the important modules you are working through over the year. Just how many themes you develop over the nursing course is something to negotiate with your personal tutor. I would not advise that you develop dozens as you need to sustain motivation, but a handful will enable you to pick up on reflections and discoveries wherever you study.

2. *Theme significance.* Next, I recommend that you include a paragraph or two stating the importance of this theme in nursing as you currently understand it, as well as your purpose in studying it. This should be entered on the same date as the theme was commenced. It will form a reminder of just how you thought about the concept at the outset of your enquiries. Later, it is often beneficial to look back on this and consider whether your insights have grown, your perspectives shifted. If we continue our example of listening, perhaps the opening purpose statement might look like this:

    Listening is vital to nursing. We cannot build a rapport with the patient until we have demonstrated that we listen to them effectively. While we need to catalogue their signs of illness, the symptoms are equally important, and these have to be heard. We have to understand how the patient perceives their circumstances. Nursing care involves planning, but this has to be shared, and patients wish to know that their perspectives are respected. Nursing care changes, and a frequent prompt for that is how the patient feels about their progress. The purpose of this enquiry is to examine how listening can be best practised, how it becomes more nuanced as insights are gained.

Activity 12.2 Critical thinking

Study now the above opening statement on the theme of listening. Why do you think that it needs both an indication of your current understanding of the concept and why you wish to follow it through within your studies in nursing?

An outline answer appears at the end of the chapter.

3. *Theme questions.* The next entry that I suggest you add to the theme within your portfolio are questions about it, those that indicate – for now – what you do not know. You can add to these questions incrementally as you proceed with your

studies, but it is a good idea to write down those that challenge you at the start of the theme. Dating your entries is very important, because as your portfolio record expands you are likely to see questions expand and change too. Typically, a theme blossoms out with more questions and queries before – over time – it starts to recede inwards, as you start to settle on explanations of what it takes to listen well. Here are some imagined questions that I might note down if I were embarking on enquiries into listening as a nursing skill:

How do we signal that we are hearing as well as listening?

How long does it take to gather the important information?

How do we reassure the other person that we are listening well?

Does the nature of that shared by the other person affect how we are meant to listen?

Is listening to professional colleagues different to listening to patients and their relatives?

4. *Episode entries.* Your next entries under the chosen theme I will call episode entries. An episode relates to a measured enquiry that you have made which relates clearly to the theme and questions in hand. We have become accustomed to thinking about episodes as reflections on care delivery (e.g. during a clinical placement), but I would encourage you to think of episodes much more broadly and to enter these incrementally, each with the date. Entries might refer to a clinical reflection, but they could relate just as easily to a role-play exercise, a workshop, a seminar or a selection of literature. The point here is that all of these learning activities are episodes in the critical thinking sense – they have focused your attention on the theme again. Episodes may come from several different modules, and indeed well beyond (e.g. a study day that you attended, a debate that you reviewed in the national press).

The entries that you are making now can be thought of as a form of musing. They capture what you thought significant to the theme in question. If they have a reflective framework format, that is fine as these too encourage you to muse. Some episodes refer directly to the questions that you raised at the start of the theme, while some others will not. Both are fine for now. The point is to record them clearly and succinctly, acknowledging 'what you think for now' and 'what you wonder about'. Episodes are your work in progress and they are a very good focus for discussions with a personal tutor. Here is my example from the listening case study:

I was involved in a workshop today, one designed to help patients manage Type 2 diabetes. The group leader convening the group reminded everyone of its purpose, and then she asked each patient in turn to describe how they had been managing their diabetes during the preceding week. Patients varied in their comfort recounting their work with diet, drugs and monitoring devices. All of the patients felt able to report highs and lows in their coping with the condition. I noticed, though, that the group leader did not dwell too much on what patients said before she invited the next contribution. It made me wonder what purpose this reporting had for the nurse, what purpose it served. Yes, it helped patients to report their experiences, but I wondered what the nurse could do with that. She did not, for example, try to solve a patient's problem there and then. She did not take notes. I asked the nurse about this afterwards and she explained that she wanted to help the patients unload a worry, feel part of the group again. But the listening purpose for her was quite distinct and instinctive. She wanted to get a feel for whether the patients were optimistic or pessimistic at present about their self-care. That, she explained, would affect the next workshop activity. I realised that there might be something called public listening which was different to listening on a one-to-one basis.

If you record an episode relating to articles or books read or a website visited, be sure to record the relevant reference details as you may need to return to them again. Notice once again, though, that this example episode is closely related to practice, that which moves towards 'how' from 'what'. My first reaction in that workshop might have been that the nurse was dismissive of the patients, but she did have a purpose for listening in that manner and it seemed valuable. There was a connection between 'how' and 'why' – I was starting to access some template thinking.

Activity 12.3   Reflection

How many episodes do you think you should record in your portfolio? Is it a case of 'the more the merrier'? Do you think you should ration the entries, or else make sure that they cover the different sources of information, clinical experience, reading, lectures, and so on?

An outline answer is given at the end of the chapter.

5. *Summing up entries.* Periodically, you will need to make a different sort of entry in your portfolio – I call these 'summing-up' entries. You have probably guessed their purpose from their name, but I do not want you to think that they only appear as the theme is closed. Within a theme, perhaps one extending over several study modules, you may have several summing-up entries to make, each dated so that you can review your thinking over time. A summing-up entry is one where you pull several strands of insight together and answer some of the questions that you posed at the start of the theme. To sum up is to take stock of your discoveries. One of the key reasons for summing-up entries is that themes can seem to explode in different directions if you do not take stock. Summing up entries, then, are about keeping your ideas together, drawing threads together from different sources of information. Does a particular researcher seem to have captured something vital about the theme, something that arose again and again in practice? Does a communication theory now seem to be missing some key ideas? To what extent could practice recommend things about listening that we have missed on campus?

Here is an extract from my case study on listening, one in which I sum up some thoughts:

I have discovered a few things. Listening is not simply a technique; there is a context to create or manage. I set the scene, choosing a quiet place for the conversation. The patient wants me to listen to something more intimate, that which worries them. But the context of conversation, how much privacy that the patient feels they have, often determines how much they reveal. It could determine how much information I have to handle. That is why I feel anxious about confidential listening. I do not know what might come out from the patient. I might not feel equal to it. But discussions with my practice supervisor remind me that I cannot promise to resolve all patient worries. I cannot remove risk, eradicate anxiety. I can only resolve some things, signal to a patient that I am trying to help. My practice supervisor has been practising for ten years, so her assessment seems realistic. But what I have been reading about listening to people from other cultures (see episode 23 January 2020) suggests that it might not be so easy to contain some patients' expectations. For some patients, to listen is to commit to putting things right. So, I have to anticipate different assumptions about the role of the nurse, self-care, or the lack of it in some traditions.

Did you notice in this extract that I have started to refer to different sorts of listening? Listening in a one-to-one context is confidential in nature, something rather different to listening in the diabetes self-help group. I am learning a template, to use listening in different ways, at different times and for different purposes.

6. *Coda entry.* Your last entry to the portfolio theme I call a coda entry. It is that which brings the theme to a close. You feel that you have progressed as far as possible with it. The majority of questions have been answered, and importantly you feel that you understand what is skilful about the use of that concept in practice. If you look back now to Tables 3.1 and 3.2 in Chapter 3, you should be operating very much towards the independent thinking end of the spectrum described there. A coda entry is likely to be rather longer than the episode entries, and in some skill-based nursing courses it might take the form of a project report or an essay. Because such an entry would be rather long, I do not offer you a listening example here, but a coda entry should offer four things:

   - *A critique of how useful information has seemed (e.g. theory, research evidence, clinical audit).* Perhaps I observe that communication theory provides descriptors for managing listening as part of a dialogue, but the nuances of listening, that which is contextual, still require some research. There is scope for a new theory of group listening, that which occurs when an audience is present.
   - *An indication of just how complex and valuable the concept or skill is.* The more private things that the patient reveals, that which is closest to their values, beliefs and fears, the more time is needed to hear what they say. At some point, listening becomes counselling, and the nurse has to be circumspect about their abilities at that point.
   - *Recognition of the 'what', 'why' and 'how' of the concept in use.* Perhaps in my coda I identify the sorts of subjects that I feel confident listening about (the 'what'). It indicates something of why it is important to allocate more listening time in particular circumstances. Perhaps it signals how

summarising patient concerns helps to signal what I have understood from the patient's account.

• *Why this concept explains and advances nursing.* Perhaps here I conclude that patients repeatedly value the nurse's listening ability as a key feature of care. Listening is a key skill for nurses in the eyes of patients that I have met.

Activity 12.4   Critical thinking

Draw breath now to consider what has been recommended above. Building some conceptual themes within your portfolio does not necessarily replace what you must record as experience (the learning log). But it does reach across modules of study, across campus and practice placement, to focus on concepts, and skills that can help to unlock how accomplished practitioners reason and work to best effect (their templates).

Imagine now that you are meeting with your personal tutor. What sort of learning issues do you think you could discuss with them using thematic portfolio entries such as these?

Some ideas are given at the end of the chapter.

Chapter summary

In this chapter, we have explored what a portfolio might include – it is both a record of work completed (the log element) and at best a proof of learning, that which demonstrates critical thinking and reflection of a high order. It is something that helps bring you closer to the sort of polished and effective template reasoning that successful registered nurses use. While the format of a portfolio may vary depending on university requirements, there remains scope to build entries that attend to the 'what', 'why' and 'how' of nursing practice.

It is through themed entries within a portfolio that you have the opportunity to combine different sorts of information and insight into questions and answers closely associated with the successful delivery of nursing care. Thematic portfolio entries need an adequate structure, and work best when developed with a tutor, but it is possible for you to learn to combine sources of information and become a quizzical thinker. In building the portfolio, it is important to carefully date entries, to return to and review what has been recorded before summing up and then making final entries on each theme.

Activities: brief outline answers

Activity 12.1 Reflection (page 188)

1. One of the problems of modular nursing courses is that they chop up learning in ways which make it harder to piece ideas back together, the *so what?* thinking that seems important in practice. Running thematic portfolio enquiries helps you to find focus in your work. Gina, for example, believed it helped that when she went on clinical placements, she knew what she was looking for. If you are already a registered nurse, the theme can help to give purpose to evidence that you collect for update learning purposes, that which enables you to revalidate your practice with the NMC (2019).

2. If you are a nursing student, the obvious person to discuss plans with is your personal tutor, but you might also show your entries to your practice supervisor or link tutor. If you are a registered nurse, then a sympathetic manager might well be an enthusiastic consultant, especially if your work also has the potential to improve service provision.

3. All of the study activities reviewed in this book have the potential to fuel your thematic entries within the portfolio, but do not limit yourselves to those. Since 2020, the Covid-19 pandemic provides a wealth of healthcare debate within the media, and this could, for example, fuel entries on cross-infection control, risk assessment and managing anxiety. Media beyond your course might provide material for reflection.

Activity 12.2 Critical thinking (page 189)

All enquiries need a starting point, a description of what you think or believe you know at the outset. You might fear that you know too little or that your thinking is misguided, but record it anyway. You should not be assessed on this, and some of the most valuable discoveries are to do with the correction of prior assumptions, the layering in of new insights. I promise you that there is the chance to feel very good about your progress. Writing down the purpose of your enquiry reminds you of what you hope to discover, master or understand. That might change over time; but if you start with a clear intention, you will have begun well.

Activity 12.3 Reflection (page 191)

I am afraid that this is a 'piece of string' question – there is no set formula for the right number of entries to make under each theme within your portfolio. In my experience, though, themes often stretch to dozens of entries over the course of a nursing degree. It is possible to major on some themes, those that might help you decide on a field of practice that you would like to specialise in later. The listening case study, for instance, could point to a career in mental health or counselling. The entries that you make can come from any source, but I do think that there should be those from both campus and practice.

Activity 12.4 Critical thinking (page 193)

Thematic entries to your portfolio enable you to discuss questions about ideas and their application to practice. They help to focus your attention on 'what', 'why' and 'how'. Gina reports that her portfolio entries in particular helped her to explore questions to do with ethics. Beyond that, though, they can help you to explore doubts about your progress, as well as whether you are doing well. A skilful personal tutor can help you to appreciate the significant shift in your reasoning, the refinement of your ideas. For that reason alone, such portfolio entries are beneficial, meeting your needs as well as any course assessment ones.

Further reading

Cooper, N. and Frain, J. (eds) (2016) *ABC of Clinical Reasoning.* Chichester: Wiley-Blackwell.

This book, written by two doctors, offers an analysis of clinical reasoning from a medical perspective. You will be heartened to realise, however, that doctors and nurses share many common concerns to ensure that practice is adequately person-centred and practical to enact. Doctors learn a great deal of scientific, technical and pharmaceutical information that requires meldling into clinical practice, so they face the same sort of theory–practice learning challenge that nurses do.

de Castillo, S.L.M. (2017) *Strategies, Techniques and Approaches to Critical Thinking: A Clinical Reasoning Workbook for Nurses*, 6th edition. Philadelphia, PA: W.B. Saunders.

This book offers an additional and largely complementary focus on the links between thinking, learning and clinical practice. We share a concern for the pragmatic and skill-based nature of nursing. Much of the text assumes a different healthcare context to that of the UK; but if you wish to extend your enquiries into what I call 'practice templates', it bears reading too.

Standing, M. (2020) *Clinical Judgement and Decision Making in Nursing*, 4th edition. London: SAGE/Learning Matters.

Mooi Standing's book on clinical judgement is the logical complement to this one on critical thinking and writing. Standing elucidates the different ways in which nurses reach clinical decisions, taking into account their experience and patient needs, as well as what I write about as 'utility concerns' (those concerning resources).

Useful websites

In this book I make regular use of YouTube video recommendations (**www.youtube.com**), and I direct you there one last time now to view two videos.

www.youtube.com/watch?v=cDDWvj_q-o8

Empathy: The Human Connection to Patient Care is a four-minute film produced by the Cleveland Clinic in 2013. Do not worry about the age of this film – some issues are timeless in nursing care. I suggest that you watch it to explore template thinking. Nurses do not simply act on clinical information; they deal with the contextual circumstances of patients too. It is critical to be empathetic, person-centred; so as you think about practice skills, it is worth asking where the person fits in. This is an unusual and powerful film that offers no narrative but captures an important focus for template thinking.

www.youtube.com/watch?v=OxKILfnHM1k

Clinical Reasoning Scenario by NorthTec, Tai Tokerau Wānanga in New Zealand from 2019 is a longer film (40 minutes), but it is valuable as it details one take on the nurse's clinical reasoning processes. This includes making a nursing diagnosis, but importantly too it acknowledges the need to focus on what represents a problem, what might ensue, and what resources are available.

Glossary of key terms

absolute thinking   A low-level form of critical thinking that admits only black or white, right or wrong, and/or good or bad explanations of issues and events. Absolute thinking suggests that the nurse has yet to appreciate how situations can be more nuanced or complex than they first seem.

academic voice   A habitual and sometimes culturally informed way of thinking about the process and purpose of learning, as well as the roles of the learner and those that support them. Tutors, for example, want the nurse to think independently, inquisitively and bravely, venturing ideas that broaden their learning. But a student might have an academic voice that is much more cautious, one that simply involves pleasing the tutor by repeating arguments already made in lectures.

argument   In formal philosophy terms, an argument is something that states a position and connects to a series of underlying premises that support it. Classically, this involves the inclusion of the word 'because' in the argument. For example, 'Patients are eager collaborators in care planning because they have a vested interest in alleviating personal anxiety and meeting their own goals.' We can begin to test this philosophically when the underpinning premises are then interrogated. For example, do all patients experience anxiety? In nursing course writing and discussion, however, the term 'argument' is more loosely used to refer to a point, that which you claim is relevant, reasonable and pertinent. Such points usually have to be supported by evidence to pass muster at assessment.

case   In academic contexts, the case is a collection of arguments that explains or defends something. For example, a case might state, 'Teaching patients is a key part of nursing practice.' This is supported by a series of arguments: 'Patients need to master self-care.' 'It is more cost-effective for patients to learn self-care.' 'Nurses are interested in supporting patients and their choices and efforts.' In an academic essay, the examiner might set a case for you to discuss, or else require you to formulate a case of your own.

citation   This refers to an acknowledged source of information within your written work. It includes details of the name(s) of the author(s) and the date of publication. Further details, such as the publisher and place of publication, are then added in the reference list at the end of your work.

cognitive intelligence   Ways of reasoning in a rational way, attending to the facts, premises and arguments. Cognitive intelligence relates to the use of logic, unpicking information in a stepwise fashion (see also **emotional intelligence**).

196

conceptualisation   A concept is a means by which we can describe a cluster of information so that it is more readily conveyed to others. For example, pain is a concept, although quite a complex one. Conceptualisation refers to the process of gathering together such concepts, perhaps from new information in practice or from what you have read. This ability to group and name phenomena is important to develop the template thinking that nurses use to deliver timely, effective and efficient care. We are able to memorise situations, needs and suitable solutions that seem pertinent to a problem.

contextual thinking   Thinking about issues, problems and needs with close reference to the context in which they arise. Contextual thinking is nuanced and considered to be a relatively high level of critical thinking.

critical theory   A philosophical and research paradigm which accepts that all knowledge is shaped in some degree by power, and that the rightful role of research is to expose inequality and advance the lot of those who are disadvantaged. Marxist and feminist researchers work in the critical theory paradigm and typically use methods such as action research (collective projects designed to change healthcare).

critical thinking   The process of analysing information and arguments in a methodical way to ascertain what is truthful, reasonable, beneficial and wise. See also my full definition on page 14 in Chapter 1.

decision-making   That element of critical thinking which signals the nurse's shift in attention or focus, which means that new work has begun. For example, the nurse completing a literature search decides that enough literature has been found. The nurse's effort then moves on to cataloguing the literature. Critical thinking without such activity is not critical at all, representing merely the accumulation of information.

declarative critical thinking   That element of reasoning which relates to our confidence that something is true, proven or viable. For the nurse to proceed with care decisions, for example, certain information has to be declared true, accepted or evident. Without the confidence to assert some facts, particular arguments, critical reasoning and new care cannot proceed.

deductive thinking   The process of testing an idea or theory. This presumes that a theory has been created in the first place. The nurse then tests it out, using research, observations in practice or discussions with professional colleagues. In practice, nurses are continuously deducing what might happen from past experience; they are also inducing ideas, creating theories to explain that which surprised them through care encounters (see also **inductive thinking**).

discourse   An account of what different parties are doing together, which is meant to give substance to the process under way. For example, a discourse on rehabilitation will describe what the nurse and patient do. It will describe their interaction (support, counselling, teaching, guidance, learning). Discourses are sometimes contested and political (e.g. different discourses on the role of the researcher and 'proper science').

emotional intelligence   Ways of reasoning that enable the nurse to quickly identify how events or stances might seem to another, to appreciate how emotions are used to help interpret experience (see also **cognitive intelligence**).

empathy   The ability to identify and have due regard for the experiences and concerns of another. Empathy involves understanding the other person's perspective without necessarily having it determine your own actions. Nurses, for example, have to be empathetic about individual patient needs but independent enough to balance those against the needs of other patients.

empirical   That which can be measured or demonstrated to another. Classically, it refers to acts, documentary accounts, or statistics relating to activities. Intentions, values and attitudes only become empirical when they are articulated through action and can be measured in that way. Nursing deals with the empirical world, but it also has to operate within a world of values, beliefs, attitudes and narratives, that which seems emotionally important in the experience of nursing care.

evidence   Information that may support a given nursing argument, stance or plan of action. Traditionally, evidence has been described as a hierarchy, with research evidence at its pinnacle (evidence-based practice). However, other forms of evidence, experience, case studies, audit information, and patient satisfaction feedback and statistics are also important evidence to plan care with.

experience   That encountered before and potentially reasoned about to formulate templates for better practice. Where experience is well articulated and critically reviewed, it can contribute to evidence supporting nursing care.

independent thinking   Thinking that involves significant imagination and innovation on the part of the nurse, sometimes described as 'thinking outside the box'. The nurse is sufficiently confident to formulate clear arguments of their own, as well as backing this up with a rationale which suggests that they are able to safely transform nursing practice.

inductive thinking   The process of creating theories or explanations to explain that which has just happened. Induction is important because nurses must constantly make sense of disparate observations and experiences. The diagnosis of a patient need or problem is arrived at incrementally through piecing together observations. This is inductive reasoning (see also **deductive thinking**).

moral justice   A series of ethical arguments about what is right, equitable, fair or just, which is used as the basis of nursing care. While nursing care might advance on the basis of evidence, it might also advance on the basis of moral practice, that which is ethical.

narrative   The storyline of thought that we rehearse to ourselves about what we are doing, why we are doing it, and what purpose it serves. For example, patients develop a narrative to explain what being a patient is, which may or may not fit with the doctor or nurse's expectation of the patient role.

naturalistic (or interpretive)   A philosophical and research paradigm that insists the only way we can authentically understand the world is by studying it in context and trusting respondents to share their experiences and meanings used in the world. The naturalistic paradigm is strongly shaped by social scientists and widely deployed in nursing as researchers explore patient experiences.

paradigm   A widely agreed way of thinking and understanding the world that holds sway over a wide range of thinkers and comes to define how the world should be seen. Thomas Kuhn observed that science moves forward through scientific revolutions, where one paradigm (explanation of the world) is replaced by another. In research, there are currently three paradigms for describing research as an activity: positivist, naturalistic and critical theory.

paraphrase   To express another's arguments within your own paper using your own words. It is critical to cite the source in the text using brackets (author's surname and date of publication). Ensure that you also clearly cite secondary sources drawn upon.

position   Within an essay, the stance that you take on a case made by others. Imagine the case states that all nurses should teach patients self-care. Two obvious stances suggest themselves, either support for or arguments against the case. But a third is also possible: 'Under XYZ circumstances, we cannot readily educate the patient' (perhaps something about the learning ability of the patient).

positivist   A paradigm of research and philosophy that focuses strongly upon the world as a place of facts, traits and dispositions, that which can be explored using the methods of the natural sciences. The emphasis of positivist research is upon carefully controlled design, namely that designed to secure valid and reliable data, as well as that which is open to replication later.

premise   A premise describes that which you accept as true, factual or demonstrable. Arguments are typically built upon premises (that which the nurse accepts as a given) and that which is reinforced by evidence. So, for example, a premise of nursing may be that we help patients to make their own decisions. This is based upon nursing as a profession that helps patients towards their own well-being. Nurses do not direct patients what to do. This sort of premise might support an argument advocating person-centred care.

reflection   The process of thinking in or upon action so as to better understand the event and to ascertain what within it requires the nurse's attention or adjustment. Reflection focuses upon our own and others' actions in order to improve working relationships. See also my full definition on page 35 in Chapter 2.

seminar   A tutor or group leader discussion where participants return with information and ideas that are designed to shed light on a mutually agreed topic. Seminars require preparation and an active engagement on the part of students, who must share their own discoveries and thinking about that found.

source   Information may come from a primary source (where it was first presented and argued) or a secondary source (where someone else has then commented upon or summarised that original information). Both require citation in an essay.

speculation   The business of supposing or imagining what is happening or required. In nursing, speculation is important – it facilitates more innovative care. The nurse must feel brave enough to speculate about what is wrong and what might help.

taxonomy   A framework to describe how different elements of a subject relate to one another, and to order them in such a way that a process is better understood. Learning, for example, can be described in terms of different levels and areas. A taxonomy (such as Bloom's) describes when learning becomes more sophisticated.

template   A predisposition to reason in a particular way. Nurses develop templates, shortcuts that help them to interpret information smoothly and quickly when dealing with, for example, anxious patients. A rigid template, however, might limit professional development or threaten patient safety. What distinguishes clinical reasoning from academic reasoning is the use of templates to address needs and problems in a real-time context, often one where there is an incomplete supply of available information. Template reasoning is pragmatic, weighing needs against resources and using experience to attend to what patients and their relatives, as well as your fellow students, might expect from an encounter. Template reasoning develops over time through paying careful attention to past episodes of care. It is, however, enhanced when nurses learn to conceptualise needs and viable solutions that have a significant chance of being both acceptable and successful. While research exists as regards the process of clinical decision-making, it remains unclear whether any prescribed set of steps can entirely capture the weighing up of information that nurses use as they rerspond to care requirements.

transitional thinking   A stage or level of thinking where the individual starts to admit the possibility that a range of factors might shape events or explain what is happening. Transitional thinking suggests that the nurse is starting to see other possibilities, to understand issues in more complex ways.

utility   That which has practical value, which is workable or usable. Not all nursing knowledge has practice utility (i.e. can be deployed at the bedside). However, knowledge may have a professional utility, being of benefit for the ways in which nurses conceive of themselves and their work.

workshop   The process of learning a subject or skill through mutual enquiries and discussion that serve to unpack what is involved. Typically, workshops are used with subjects where there is no perfect or absolutely correct best practice. So, for example, a listening workshop might be convened in association with the support of dying patients. Participants try out explanations of what they are doing while listening; they speculate about what is beneficial or desirable.

References

Adams, L. (2016) *Learning a New Skill Is Easier Said Than Done*. Available at: www.gordontraining.com/free-workplace-articles/learning-a-new-skill-is-easier-said-than-done/

Adams, M.B., Kaplan, B., Sobko, H.J., Kuziemsky, C., Ravvaz, K. and Koppel, R. (2015) Learning from colleagues about healthcare IT implementation and optimization: lessons from a medical informatics listserv. *Journal of Medical Systems*, 39(1): 157–62.

Ahmad, Z., Anderson, J., Bissoondatt, J., Campbell, P., Dhaliwal, T., Dhami, G., et al. (2018) A phenomenological analysis of the experience of nursing students' usage of various technologies within a hybrid degree program. *Canadian Journal of Nursing Informatics*, 13(2). Available at: http:/tinyurl.com/y4ohqkew

Aleshire, M.E., Dampier, A. and Woltenberg, L. (2019) Evaluating undergraduate nursing students' attitudes toward health care teams in the context of an interprofessionally-focused nursing course. *Journal of Professional Nursing*, 35(1): 37–43.

Alfayoumi, I. (2019) The impact of combining concept-based learning and concept-mapping pedagogies on nursing students' clinical reasoning abilities. *Nurse Education Today*, 72: 40–6.

Allen, D. (2015) *The Invisible Work of Nurses: Hospitals, Organisation and Healthcare*. London: Routledge.

Anderson, L.W. and Krathwohl, D.R. (eds) (2001) *A Taxonomy for Learning, Teaching, and Assessing: A Revision of Bloom's Taxonomy of Educational Objectives*. Boston, MA: Pearson.

Andrew, L., Ewens, B.A. and Maslin-Prothero, S. (2015) Enhancing the online learning experience using virtual interactive classrooms. *Australian Journal of Advanced Nursing*, 32(4): 22–31.

Aydin Er, R., Sehiralti, M. and Akpinar, A. (2017) Attributes of a good nurse: the opinions of nursing students. *Nursing Ethics*, 24(2): 238–50.

Barratt, J. (2019) Developing clinical reasoning and effective communication skills in advanced practice. *Nursing Standard*, 34(2): 37–44.

Baxter Magolda, M.B. (1992) *Knowing and Reasoning in College: Gender-Related Patterns in Students' Intellectual Development*. San Francisco, CA: Jossey-Bass.

Baylis, D. (2015) How to avoid negligence claims. *Practice Nurse*, 45(1): 10–11.

Bifarin, O. and Stonehouse, D. (2017) Clinical supervision: an important part of every nurse's practice. *British Journal of Nursing*, 26(6): 331–5.

Blomberg, K., Lindqvist, O., Werkander Harstäde, C., Söderman, A. and Östlund, U. (2019) Translating the Patient Dignity Inventory. *International Journal of Palliative Care,* 25(7): 334–43.

Bloom, B. (ed.) (1956) *Taxonomy of Educational Objectives: The Classification of Educational Goals.* New York: David McKay.

Blum, C.A. (2018) Does podcast use enhance critical thinking in nursing education? *Nursing Education Perspectives,* 39(2): 91–3.

Bolton, G. and Delderfield, R. (2018) *Reflective Practice: Writing and Professional Development,* 5th edition. London: SAGE.

Bolton, J.W. (2015) Varieties of clinical reasoning. *Journal of Evaluative Clinical Practice,* 21(3): 486–9.

Buckley, C., McCormack, B. and Ryan, A. (2018) Working in a storied way: narrative-based approaches to person-centred care and practice development in older adult residential care settings. *Journal of Clinical Nursing,* 27(5–6) e858–72.

Calhoun, E.A. and Esparza, A. (eds) (2017) *Patient Navigation: Overcoming Borders to Care.* New York: Springer.

Canniford, L.J. and Fox-Young, S. (2015) Learning and assessing competence in reflective practice: student evaluation of the relative value of aspects of an integrated, interactive reflective practice syllabus. *Collegian,* 22(3): 291–7.

Carr, V.L., Sangiorgi, D., Büscher, M., Junginger, S. and Cooper, R. (2011) Integrating evidence-based design and experience-based approaches in healthcare service design. *HERD,* 4(4): 12–33.

Casey, M., Cooney, A., O'Connell, R., Hegarty, J.-M., Brady, A.-M., O'Reilly, P., et al. (2017) Nurses', midwives' and key stakeholders' experiences and perceptions on requests to demonstrate the maintenance of professional competence. *Journal of Advanced Nursing,* 73(3): 653–64.

Cavallazzi, R., Saad, M. and Marik, P.E. (2012) Delirium in the ICU: an overview. *Annals of Intensive Care,* 2(49): 1–11.

Chatfield, T. (2018) *Critical Thinking: Your Guide to Effective Argument, Successful Analysis and Independent Study.* London: SAGE.

Compton, R.M., Owilli, A.O., Norlin, E.E. and Hubbard Murdoch, N.L. (2020) Does problem-based learning in nursing education empower learning? *Nurse Education in Practice,* 44. doi: 10.1016/nepr.2020.102752

Conroy, T. (2018) Factors influencing the delivery of the fundamentals of care: perceptions of nurses, nursing leaders and healthcare consumers. *Journal of Clinical Nursing,* 27(11–12): 2373–86.

Cooper, N. and Frain, J. (eds) (2016) *ABC of Clinical Reasoning.* Chichester: Wiley-Blackwell.

Creswell, J.W. and Creswell, J.D. (2018) *Research Design: Qualitative, Quantitative, and Mixed Methods Approaches,* 5th edition. London: SAGE.

Cui, J., Li, F. and Shi, Z.-L. (2019) Origin and evolution of pathogenic coronaviruses. *Nature Reviews Microbiology*, 17(3): 181–92.

Cummings, L. (2016) *Case Studies in Communication Disorders*. Cambridge: Cambridge University Press.

de Castillo, S.L.M. (2017) *Strategies, Techniques and Approaches to Critical Thinking: A Clinical Reasoning Workbook for Nurses*, 6th edition. Philadelphia, PA: W.B. Saunders.

Dickson, E.A., Jones, K.I. and Lund, J.N. (2016) Skype: a platform for remote, interactive skills instruction. *Medical Education*, 50(11): 1151–2.

Edmonds, W.A. and Kennedy, T.D. (2016) *An Applied Guide to Research Designs: Quantitive, Qualitative, and Mixed Methods*, 2nd edition. London: SAGE.

Edwards, S. (2017) Reflecting differently. New dimensions: reflection-before-action and reflection-beyond-action. *International Practice Development Journal*, 7(1): 1–14.

Ellis, P. (2019) *Evidence-Based Practice in Nursing*, 4th edition. London: SAGE/Learning Matters.

Esterhuizen, P. (2019) *Reflective Practice in Nursing*, 4th edition. London: SAGE/Learning Matters.

Farne, H., Norris-Cervetto, E. and Warbeck-Smith, J. (2015) *Oxford Cases in Medicine and Surgery*, 2nd edition. Oxford: Oxford University Press.

Fasbender, U., Van der Heijden, B.I.J.M. and Grimshaw, S. (2018) Job satisfaction, job stress and nurses' turnover intentions: the moderating roles of on-the-job and off-the-job embeddedness. *Journal of Advanced Nursing*, 75(2): 327–37.

Fealy, G., Hegarty, J.-M., McNamara M., Casey, M., O'Leary, D., Kennedy, C., et al. (2018) Discursive constructions of professional identity in policy and regulatory discourse. *Journal of Advanced Nursing*, 74(9): 2157–66.

Feeney, Á. and Everett, S. (2020) *Understanding Supervision and Assessment in Nursing*. London: SAGE.

Flyverbom, M. (2019) *The Digital Prism: Transparency and Managed Visibilities in a Datafied World*. Cambridge: Cambridge University Press.

Freeborn, D. and Knafl, K. (2014) Growing up with cerebral palsy: perceptions of the influence of family. *Child: Care, Health and Development*, 40(5): 671–9.

Friberg, E. (2019) *Conceptual Foundations: The Bridge to Professional Nursing Practice*, 7th edition. St Louis, MO: Elsevier Mosby.

Gambrill, E. and Gibbs, L. (2017) *Critical Thinking for Helping Professionals: A Skills-Based Workbook*, 4th edition. Oxford: Oxford University Press.

Garrett, B.M. (2016) New sophistry: self-deception in the nursing academy. *Nursing Philosophy*, 17(3): 182–93.

George, A., Oluwafemi, S.O. and Joseph, B. (eds) (2017) *Holistic Healthcare: Possibilities and Challenges*. New York: Apple Academic Press.

Gibbs, G. (1988) *Learning by Doing: A Guide to Teaching and Learning Methods.* Oxford: Oxford Polytechnic Further Education Unit.

Gobet, F. (2005) Chunking models of expertise: implications for education. *Applied Cognitive Psychology,* 19(2): 183–204.

Gobet, F. and Chassy, P. (2008) Towards an alternative to Benner's theory of expert intuition in nursing: a discussion paper. *International Journal of Nursing Studies,* 45(1): 129–39.

Gold, A.L., Shechner, T., Farber, M.J., Spiro, C.N., Leibenluft, E., Pine, D.S., et al. (2016) Amygdala-corticol connectivity: associations with anxiety, development, and threat. *Depression and Anxiety,* 33(10): 917–26.

Goldsberry, J.W. (2018) Advanced practice nurses leading the way: interprofessional collaboration. *Nurse Education Today,* 65: 1–3.

Grace, P.J. (2017) *Nursing Ethics and Professional Responsibility in Advanced Practice,* 3rd edition. London: Jones & Bartlett Learning.

Grant, A., McKimm, J. and Murphy, F. (2017) *Developing Reflective Practice: A Guide for Medical Students, Doctors and Teachers.* Chichester: Wiley-Blackwell.

Greetham, B. (2018) *How to Write Better Essays,* 4th edition. London: Palgrave Macmillan.

Grigorescu, S., Cazan, A.-M., Grigorescu, O.D. and Rogozea, L.M. (2018) The role of the personality traits and work characteristics in the prediction of the burnout syndrome among nurses: a new approach within predictive, preventive, and personalized medicine concept. *EPMA Journal,* 9(4): 355–65.

Grob, R., Schlesinger, M., Parker, A.M., Shaller, D., Barre, L.R., Martino, S.C., et al. (2016) Breaking narrative ground: innovative methods for rigorously eliciting and assessing patient narratives. *Health Services Research,* 51(S2): 1248–72.

Haines, K.J., Savin, C.M., Hibbert, E., Boehm, L.M., Aparanji, K., Bakhru, R.N., et al. (2019) Key mechanisms by which post-ICU activities can improve in-ICU care: results of the international THRIVE collaboratives. *Intensive Care Medicine,* 45(7): 939–47.

Hanscomb, S. (2016) *Critical Thinking: The Basics.* London: Routledge.

Hashemiparast, M., Negarandeh, R. and Theofanidis, D. (2019) Exploring the barriers of utilizing theoretical knowledge in clinical settings: a qualitative study. *International Journal of Nursing Sciences,* 6(4): 399–405.

Hayhurst, C.J., Pandharipande, P.P. and Hughes, C.G. (2016) Intensive care unit delirium: a review of diagnosis, prevention, and treatment. *Anesthesiology,* 125(6): 1229–41.

Heinrich, P. (2017) *When Role Play Comes Alive: A Theory and Practice.* London: Palgrave Macmillan.

Higgs, J., Jensen, G.M., Loftus, S. and Christensen, N. (2019) *Clinical Reasoning in the Health Professions,* 4th edition. Edinburgh: Elsevier.

Hingston, K. and Cross, R.M. (2017) Preceptor masterclass in the emergency department: improving the experience for undergraduate nursing supervision. *Australian Nursing & Midwifery Journal,* 25(1): 41.

Holloway, I. and Galvin, K. (2016) *Qualitative Research in Nursing and Healthcare.* Chichester: Wiley-Blackwell.

Honey, P. and Mumford, A. (1982) *The Manual of Learning Styles.* London: Peter Honey.

Hong, S. and Yu, P. (2017) Comparison of the effectiveness of two styles of case-based learning implemented in lectures for developing nursing students' critical thinking ability: a randomized controlled trial. *International Journal of Nursing Studies,* 68: 16–24.

Hutchinson, M., Hurley, J., Kozlowski, D. and Whitehair, L. (2017) The use of emotional intelligence capabilities in clinical reasoning and decision-making: a qualitative, exploratory study. *Journal of Clinical Nursing,* 27(3–4): e600–10.

Hyde-Wyatt, J.P. (2014) Managing hyperactive delirium and spinal immobilisation in the intensive care setting: a case study and reflective discussion of the literature. *Intensive and Critical Care Nursing,* 30(3): 138–44.

Jenicek, M. (2018) *How to Think in Medicine: Reasoning, Decision Making, and Communication in Health Sciences and Professions.* London: Productivity Press.

Jessee, M.A. (2018) Pursuing improvement in clinical reasoning: the integrated clinical education theory. *Journal of Nursing Education,* 57(1): 7–13.

Jordan, A. and Chambers, C. (2017) Meeting the needs of families: facilitating access to credible healthcare information. *Evidence-Based Nursing,* 20(1): 2–4.

Kaihlanen, A.M., Haavisto, E., Strandell-Laine, C. and Salminen, L. (2018) Facilitating the transition from a nursing student to a registered nurse in the final clinical practicum: a scoping literature review. *Scandinavian Journal of Caring Sciences,* 32(2): 466–77.

Kavanagh, J.M. and Szweda, C. (2017) A crisis in competency: the strategic and ethical imperative to assessing new graduate nurses' clinical reasoning. *Nursing Education Perspectives,* 38(2): 57–62.

Kelsey, C. and Hayes, S. (2015) Frameworks and models: scaffolding or strait jackets? Problematising reflective practice. *Nurse Education in Practice,* 15(6): 393–6.

Kitson, A., Brook A., Harvey, G., Jordan, Z., Marshall, R., O'Shea, R., et al. (2018) Using complexity and network concepts to inform healthcare knowledge translation. *International Journal of Health Policy and Management,* 7(3): 231–43.

Ko, L.N., Rana, J. and Burgin, S. (2019) Teaching & learning tips 5: making lectures more 'active'. *International Journal of Dermatology,* 57(3): 351–4.

Koivisto, J.-M., Multisilta, J., Niemi, H., Katajisto, J. and Eriksson, E. (2016) Learning by playing: a cross-sectional descriptive study of nursing students' experiences of learning clinical reasoning. *Nurse Education Today,* 45: 22–8.

Kuhn, T.S. (2012) *The Structure of Scientific Revolutions,* 50th anniversary edition. Chicago, IL: University of Chicago Press.

Lai, C.-Y. and Wu, C.-C. (2016) Promoting nursing students' clinical learning through a mobile e-portfolio. *Computers, Informatics, Nursing,* 34(11): 535–43.

Lee, J.J., Clarke, C.L. and Carson, M.N. (2018) Nursing students' learning dynamics and influencing factors in clinical contexts. *Nurse Education in Practice,* 29: 103–9.

Lee, K.-C., Yu, C.-C., Hsieh, P.-L., Li, C.-C. and Chao, Y.-F.C. (2018) Situated teaching improves empathy learning of the students in a BSN program: a quasi-experimental study. *Nurse Education Today*, 64: 138–43.

Linsley, P., Kane, R. and Barker, J. (2019) *Evidence-Based Practice for Nurses and Healthcare Professionals*, 4th edition. London: SAGE.

Littlejohn, A. and Hood, N. (2018) *Reconceptualizing Learning in the Digital Age: The (Un)democratising Potential of MOOCs*. New York: Springer.

Lovatt, A. (2014) Defining critical thoughts. *Nurse Education Today*, 34(5): 670–2.

Magnusson, J. and Zackariasson, M. (2018) Student independence in undergraduate projects: different understandings in different academic contexts. *Journal of Further and Higher Education*, 43(10): 1404–19.

Mangubat, M.D.B. (2017) Emotional intelligence: five pieces to the puzzle. *Nursing2020*, 47(7): 51–3.

Marx, E.W. and Padmanabhan, P. (2020) *Healthcare Digital Transformation: How Consumerism, Technology and Pandemic Are Accelerating the Future*. London: Routledge.

Mason, C.H. (2005) Addressing complex health issues: developing contextual knowing through sequenced writing and presentations. *International Journal of Nursing Education Scholarship*, 2(1). doi: 10.2202/1548-923x.1149

McBee, E., Ratcliffe, T., Schuwirth, L., O'Neill, D., Meyer, H., Madden, S.J., et al. (2018) Context and clinical reasoning: understanding the medical student perspective. *Perspectives on Medical Education*, 7(4): 256–63.

McCarthy, B., McCarthy, J., Trace, A. and Grace, P. (2018) Addressing ethical concerns arising in nursing and midwifery students' reflective assignments. *Nursing Ethics*, 25(6): 773–85.

McKinnon, J. (2018) In their shoes: an ontological perspective on empathy in nursing practice. *Journal of Clinical Nursing*, 27(21–2): 3882–93.

McLeod, S. (2020) *Correlation Definitions, Examples and Interpretation*. Available at: www.simplypsychology.org/correlation.html

McPherson, F. (2018) *Effective Notetaking*, 3rd edition. Wellington: Wayz Press.

Merisier, S., Larue, C. and Boyer, L. (2018) How does questioning influence nursing students' clinical reasoning in problem-based learning? A scoping review. *Nurse Education Today*, 65: 108–15.

Monrouxe, L.V. and Rees, C.E. (2017) *Healthcare Professionalism: Improving Practice Through Reflections on Workplace Dilemmas*. Chichester: Wiley-Blackwell.

Morgan, R. (2019) Using seminars as a teaching method in undergraduate nurse education. *British Journal of Nursing*, 28(6): 374–6.

Murphy, C.-A. (2019) The limits of evidence and the implications of context: considerations when implementing pathways to intervention for children with language disorders. *International Journal of Language & Communication Disorders*, 54(1): 20–3.

Nelson-Brantley, H.V., David Bailey, K., Batcheller, J., Bernard, N., Caramanica, L. and Snow, F. (2019) Grassroots to global: the future of nursing leadership. *JONA The Journal of Nursing Administration*, 49(3): 118–20.

Nursing and Midwifery Council (NMC) (2018a) *The Code: Professional Standards of Practice and Behaviour for Nurses, Midwives and Nursing Associates.* Available at: www.nmc.org.uk/globalassets/sitedocuments/nmc-publications/nmc-code.pdf

Nursing and Midwifery Council (NMC) (2018b) *Future Nurse: Standards of Proficiency for Registered Nurses.* Available at: www.nmc.org.uk/globalassets/sitedocuments/education-standards/future-nurse-proficiencies.pdf

Nursing and Midwifery Council (NMC) (2019) *Revalidation.* Available at: www.nmc.org.uk/globalassets/sitedocuments/revalidation/how-to-revalidate-booklet.pdf

Odell, M. (2015) Detection and management of the deteriorating ward patient: an evaluation of nursing practice. *Journal of Clinical Nursing*, 24(1–2): 173–82.

Oermann, M.H., De Gagne, J.C. and Phillips, B.C. (eds) (2018) *Teaching in Nursing and Role of the Educator: The Complete Guide to Best Practice in Teaching, Evaluation, and Curriculum Development*, 2nd edition. New York: Springer.

Oriot, D. and Alinier, G. (2018) *Pocket Book for Simulation Debriefing in Healthcare.* London: Springer.

Page, K. and McKinney, A. (eds) (2012) *Nursing the Acutely Ill Adult: Case Book.* Milton Keynes: Open University Press.

Pape, S. (2019) *Being Right: A Beginner's Guide to Logical Fallacies and Deductive Reasoning*, 4th edition. Independently published.

Pears, R. and Shields, G. (2019) *Cite Them Right: The Essential Referencing Guide*, 11th edition. London: Red Globe Press.

Peddle, M., Jokwiro, Y., Carter, M. and Young, T. (2016) A professional portfolio of learning for undergraduate nursing students. *Australian Nursing & Midwifery Journal*, 24(4): 40.

Pickles, D., de Lacey, S. and King, L. (2019) Conflict between nursing student's personal beliefs and professional nursing values. *Nursing Ethics*, 26(4): 1087–100.

Presti, C.R. (2019) Peer learning and role-play to enhance critical thinking. *Nurse Educator*, 44(1): 33.

Price, B. (1990) *Body Image: Nursing Concepts and Care.* London: Prentice Hall.

Price, B. (2003) Academic voices and the challenges of tutoring. *Nurse Education Today*, 23(8): 628–37.

Price, B. (2014) Avoiding plagiarism: guidance for nursing students. *Nursing Standard*, 28(26): 45–51.

Price, B. (2016) Enabling patients to manage altered body image. *Nursing Standard*, 31(16–18): 60–71.

Price, B. (2017) How to write a reflective practice case study. *Primary Health Care*, 27(9): 35–42.

Price, B. (2019a) How to make clear and compelling written arguments: advice for nurses. *Primary Health Care*, 29(6): 36–42.

Price, B. (2019b) *Delivering Person-Centred Care in Nursing*. London: SAGE/Learning Matters.

Ray-Barruel, G., Woods, C., Larsen, E.N., Marsh, N., Ullman, A.J. and Rickard, C.M. (2019) Nurses' decision-making about intravenous administration set replacement: a qualitative study. *Journal of Clinical Nursing*, 28(21–22): 3786–95.

Roberts, M. (2015) *Critical Thinking and Writing for Mental Health Nursing Students*. London: SAGE/Learning Matters.

Rodgers, B.L., Jacelon, C.S. and Knafl, K.A. (2018) Concept analysis and the advance of nursing knowledge: state of the science. *Journal of Nursing Scholarship*, 50(4): 451–9.

Rolfe, G., Jasper, M. and Freshwater, D. (2011) *Critical Reflection in Practice: Generating Knowledge for Care*, 2nd edition. London: Palgrave Macmillan.

Ryan, C.L. and McAllister, M.M. (2020) Professional development in clinical teaching: an action research study. *Nurse Education Today*, 85: 104306. doi: 10.1016/j.nedt.2019.104306

Ryan, G. (2018) Introduction to positivism, interpretivism and critical theory. *Nurse Researcher*, 25(4): 14–20.

Sala, G. and Gobet, F. (2017) Experts' memory superiority for domain-specific random material generalizes across fields of expertise: a meta-analysis. *Memory & Cognition*, 45: 183–93.

Salifu, D.A., Gross, J., Salifu, M.A. and Ninnoni, J.P.K. (2019) Experiences and perceptions of the theory-practice gap in nursing in a resource-constrained setting: a qualitative description study. *Nursing Open*, 6(1): 72–83.

Sasaki, T., Sato, T., Nakai, Y., Sasahira, N., Isayama, H. and Koike, K. (2019) Brain metastasis in pancreatic cancer: two case reports. *Medicine (Baltimore)*, 98(4): e14227.

Schober, M. (2019) An international perspective of advanced nursing practice. In P. McGee and C. Inman (eds), *Advanced Practice in Healthcare: Dynamic Developments in Nursing and Allied Health Professions*. Chichester: Wiley-Blackwell, pp20–38.

Schön, D.A. (1987) *Educating the Reflective Practitioner: Toward a New Design for Teaching and Learning in the Professions*. San Francisco, CA: Jossey-Bass.

Shakeel, A.K. and Bhatti, R. (2018) Semantic web and ontology-based application for digital libraries: an investigation from LIS professionals in Pakistan. *The Electronic Library*, 36(5): 826–41.

Sinclair, S., Beamer, K., Hack, T.F., McClement, S., Raffin Bouchal, S., Chochinov, H.M., et al. (2016) Sympathy, empathy, and compassion: a grounded theory study of palliative care patients' understandings, experiences, and preferences. *Palliative Medicine*, 31(5): 437–47.

Skela-Savič, B., Hvalič-Touzery, S. and Pesjak, K. (2017) Professional values and competencies as explanatory factors for the use of evidence-based practice in nursing. *Journal of Advanced Nursing*, 73(8): 1910–23.

Smith, J.A. and Judd, J. (2020) COVID-19: vulnerability and the power of privilege in a pandemic. *Health Promotion Journal of Australia*, 31(2): 158–60.

Smith, P.K., Cowie, H. and Blades, M. (2015) *Understanding Children's Development*, 6th edition. Chichester: Wiley-Blackwell.

Sokol, D. (2018) *Tough Choices: Stories from the Front Line of Medical Ethics.* London: Book Guild.

Standing, M. (2020) *Clinical Judgement and Decision Making in Nursing*, 4th edition. London: SAGE/Learning Matters.

Steele, W. (2020) *Reducing Compassion Fatigue, Secondary Traumatic Stress, and Burnout: A Trauma-Sensitive Workbook.* London: Routledge.

Stojan, J.N., Clay, M.A. and Lypson, M.L. (2016) Assessing patient-centred care through direct observation of clinical encounters. *BMJ Quality & Safety*, 25(3): 135–7.

Sundler, A.J., Blomberg, K., Bisholt, B., Eklund, A., Windahl, J. and Larsson, M. (2019) Experiences of supervision during clinical education among specialised nursing students in Sweden: a cross-sectional study. *Nurse Education Today*, 79: 20–4.

Takase, M., Niitani, M., Imai, M. and Okada, M. (2019) Students' perceptions of teaching factors that demotivate their learning in lectures and laboratory-based skills practice. *International Journal of Nursing Sciences*, 6(4): 414–20.

Thompson, S. and Thompson, N. (2018) *The Critically Reflective Practitioner*, 2nd edition. London: Palgrave Macmillan.

Trocky, N.M. and Buckley, K.M. (2016) Evaluating the impact of wikis on student learning: an integrative review. *Journal of Professional Nursing*, 32(5): 364–76.

Tuomikoski, A.-M., Ruotsalainen, H., Mikkonen, K., Miettunen, J. and Kääriäinen, M. (2018) The competence of nurse mentors in mentoring students in clinical practice: a cross-sectional study. *Nurse Education Today*, 71: 78–83.

Vae, K.J.U., Engström, M., Mårtensson, G. and Löfmark, A. (2018) Nursing students' and preceptors' experience of assessment during clinical practice: a multilevel repeated-interview study of student-preceptor dyads. *Nurse Education in Practice*, 30: 13–19.

Vincent, C. and Amalberti, R. (2016) *Safer Healthcare: Strategies for the Real World.* New York: Springer.

Vinson, A.H. (2016) 'Constrained collaboration': patient empowerment discourse as resource for countervailing power. *Sociology of Health & Illness*, 38(8): 1364–78.

Wallace, M. and Wray, A. (2016) *Critical Reading and Writing for Postgraduates*, 3rd edition. London: SAGE.

Weaver, C.B., Kane-Gill, S.L., Gunn, S.R., Levent, K. and Smithburger, P.L. (2017) A retrospective analysis of the effectiveness of antipsychotics in the treatment of ICU delirium. *Journal of Critical Care*, 41: 234–9.

Whitman, J.C., Zhao, J. and Todd, R.M. (2017) Alternation between different types of evidence attenuates judgments of severity. *PLoS ONE*, 12(7): e0180585.

References

Wilson, B., Woollands, A. and Barrett, D. (2019) *Care Planning: A Guide for Nurses,* 3rd edition. London: Routledge.

Wolff, M., Wagner, M.J., Poznanski, S., Schiller, J. and Santen, S. (2015) Not another boring lecture: engaging learners with active learning techniques. *Journal of Emergency Medicine,* 48(1): 85–93.

Zahavi, D. and Martiny, K. (2019) Phenomenology in nursing studies: new perspectives. *International Journal of Nursing Studies,* 93: 155–62.

Index

Note: References in *italics* are to figures, those in **bold** to tables; 'g' refers to the Glossary.